Political Violence, Armed Conflict, and Youth Adjustment

E. Mark Cummings · Christine E. Merrilees
Laura K. Taylor · Christina F. Mondi

Political Violence, Armed Conflict, and Youth Adjustment

A Developmental Psychopathology
Perspective on Research and Intervention

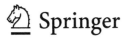 Springer

E. Mark Cummings
Department of Psychology
University of Notre Dame
Notre Dame, IN
USA

Laura K. Taylor
School of Psychology
Queens University Belfast
Belfast
UK

Christine E. Merrilees
Department of Psychology
State University of New York at Geneseo
Geneseo, NY
USA

Christina F. Mondi
Institute of Child Development
University of Minnesota
Minneapolis, MN
USA

ISBN 978-3-319-51582-3   ISBN 978-3-319-51583-0   (eBook)
DOI 10.1007/978-3-319-51583-0

Library of Congress Control Number: 2016961303

Printed on acid-free paper

This Springer imprint is published by Springer Nature
The registered company is Springer International Publishing AG
The registered company address is: Gewerbestrasse 11, 6330 Cham, Switzerland

Preface

Over one billion children are growing up throughout the world in contexts of political violence and armed conflict. A burgeoning literature attests to the significant and many risks and challenges these environments pose to the development of children. The well-being and mental health of these children are a matter of great international concern and an issue of rapidly growing interest to scholars, students, and practitioners who may wish to contribute to both understanding of the risks and challenges and the development of more effective prevention and intervention strategies to help the children cope with these environments.

However, gaining access to the contributions of this fast-growing literature involving many regions of the world presents many obstacles to those who may want to comprehend the status of what we know at this point. For example, the pertinent literature is published across multiple disciplines and in many different publication outlets, involving diverse regions of the world, so that the process of locating and evaluating this work poses daunting, even overwhelming, roadblocks for potentially interested readers. In addition, the quality of this literature is highly variable, ranging from well-intentioned but relatively weakly designed works that may not be amenable to confident interpretation to other studies that meet relatively high, even laudable, standards of methodological rigor, analysis, and interpretation.

The goal of this volume is to accomplish an accessible, up-to-date presentation and analysis of this diverse, important literature on the risks, well-being, and adjustment of children growing up throughout the world in contexts of political violence and armed conflict, including basic and applied research on these questions. Another goal is to provide an organizational framework that fosters a systematic analysis of the quality of the research. This is broadly accomplished by the application of a developmental psychopathology perspective that provides a cutting-edge basis for evaluating and fostering the study of normal development and the development of psychopathology in children.

Specifically, a four-tiered framework informed by the tenets of developmental psychopathology is employed for integrating and evaluating the current empirical literature on this topic. Although we inevitably exclude many studies from further consideration for not meeting our minimal standards of scientific rigor, beyond that, we endeavor to represent at least in the frequency counts for research, all studies that meet threshold for making contributions to the field at each tier. Notably, research on this topic poses great methodological, practical, financial, and statistical challenges. Our perspective is much work makes important contributions, even if not meeting all the criteria ideal in laboratory studies or in less challenging social-ecological contexts, so we endeavor in this book to be inclusive.

In terms of the organization of this volume, the urgency of the study of youth in contexts of political violence and armed conflict from a worldwide perspective is discussed in Chap. 1. Next, the guiding model for review in terms of a developmental psychopathology perspective is succinctly described in Chap. 2. More specifically, a framework for review of research from a developmental psychopathology perspective in terms of a four-tiered framework is presented in Chap. 3. This four-tiered "pyramid" model, which is shown in Fig. 3.1, reflects the assumption that research progresses up the pyramid in the following stages (1) the documentation of the developmental outcomes of exposure to violence, including level of exposure to traumatic violence and exploration of variations as a function of demographic differences; (2) studies additionally providing initial exploration of the role of mediators, moderators, and social-ecological contexts based on cross-sectional studies; (3) longitudinal, process-oriented work; and (4) prevention and intervention research.

For each tier, in the chapters that follow, the count of studies in the literature meeting criteria for each tier is indicated, and bottom-line messages of the research are reviewed. Given the extensive numbers of studies meeting criteria for each tier (especially Tiers 1 and 2), and the aim to accomplish a worldwide review across multiple contexts of conflict and violence that is our goal, the presentation of all studies meeting criteria, along with details on research design and social-ecological contexts, was not feasible. Accordingly, rich detail on the state of the art for each tier of research is accomplished through detailed presentations (e.g., region sampled, assessment timing, participants sampled, measures, and major findings) for a selected, substantial number of the best studies by our assessment for each tier (typically about 20 studies for each tier). The aim is to provide an extensive overview of the specific characteristics and contributions of many of the best studies at each level of analysis, all of which we judged as highly important in multiple respects. This approach is intended to provide interested students and scholars with a handy, conceptually organized reference or handbook of the characteristics, contents, and contributions of many of the specific, state-of-the-art studies that have been conducted throughout the world pertinent to each region of the world and tier of approach. We realize that we inevitably were not able to include all of the relevant studies. However, we feel confident we have accomplished an extensive representation of the state of the art in this volume that can serve as a ready and accessible handbook and reference for students and scholars interested in a review and critical analysis of this highly important, burgeoning area of study.

In addition, through the mechanism of this framework, the state of knowledge in this area is evaluated and critical assessments are made of the strengths and weaknesses of current research. We recognize that there are many practical, methodological, and statistical challenges associated with studying children's development in contexts of political violence and armed conflict. Aims of this book also include providing specific bases for advancing the state of basic, process-oriented research that examines youth adjustment at multiple social-ecological levels, including advanced concepts for stronger research design and analysis, as well as more effective, theory-guided translational prevention and intervention efforts.

Accordingly, Chap. 8 provides a vision for future research from a developmental psychopathology perspective. Recommendations are made for research at each specific tier of the "pyramid" for research on political violence, armed conflict, and youth adjustment from a developmental psychopathology perspective on research and intervention. Numerous issues and questions unresolved by current research are identified, and future directions for more integrated process-oriented basic and applied research are outlined. A central theme for future research is that translational efforts for the development of more effective and scientifically rigorous prevention and intervention research must include a closer interplay between basic and applied research that elevates the state of knowledge, increasing the likelihood that applied programs make a positive impact in the lives of children and families.

Chapter 9 concludes the book by reiterating the key messages of the road map provided by this volume for future research in this area. In particular, the road map indicates the need to expand the range of analyzed outcomes and levels of the social ecology that are examined, as well as new and more rigorous approaches toward evaluating explanatory processes accounting for the developmental outcomes in children growing up in the contexts of political violence and armed conflict. In conclusion, this volume is intended to encourage researchers to advance programs of research that are informed by developmental theory, basic and applied research, and that employ adequately sophisticated research designs and statistical methods to address the core challenges, stresses, concerns and possible sources of protection and resilience related to the normal development and development of psychopathology in children growing up in contexts fraught by political violence and armed conflict.

Notre Dame, USA   E. Mark Cummings
Geneseo, USA   Christine E. Merrilees
Belfast, UK   Laura K. Taylor
Minneapolis, USA   Christina F. Mondi

Acknowledgements

E. Mark Cummings, Christine E. Merrilees, and Laura K. Taylor were supported by awards from the National Institutes of Health (R01 HD046933) and from the Office of the First Minister & Deputy First Minister, Government of Northern Ireland (ID#2110018224).

Christina F. Mondi was supported by the National Science Foundation Graduate Research Fellowship (Grant No. 00039202). Any opinion, findings, and conclusions or recommendations expressed in this material are those of the authors and do not necessarily reflect the views of the National Science Foundation.

Contents

1   **Political Violence, Armed Conflict, and Youth Adjustment:**
    A Worldwide Perspective 1
    Defining Political Violence and Armed Conflict 2
    The Urgency of the Study of Youth 3
    References. 4

2   **Developmental Psychopathology as a Guiding Model**. 7
    Fostering Cogent Scientific Bases for Prevention and Intervention:
    Translational Research 8
    References. 9

3   **A Framework: Review of Research from a Developmental**
    Psychopathology Perspective 11
    Methodology: Search Strategy for Identifying Tier 1–3 Studies 13
    References. 15

4   **Tier 1 Studies: Documenting the Impact on Youth** 17
    Historic Research 17
    Recent Studies. 19
    Youth Outcomes 19
    Summary. 29
    References. 30

5   **Tier 2: Cross-Sectional Studies of Mediators, Process-Oriented**
    Moderators, and Social-Ecological Contexts 35
    Investigating Multiple Levels of the Social Ecology 35
    Summary. 52
    References. 53

6 **Tier 3: Longitudinal Studies of Mediators, Moderators,**
   and Multiple Social-Ecological Levels   57
   A Process-Oriented, Social-Ecological Perspective   57
   Summary...   76
   References...   77

7 **Tier 4: Prevention and Intervention Research**   81
   Summary...   93
   References...   94

8 **A Vision for Future Research from a Developmental**
   Psychopathology Perspective   97
   References...   105

9 **Conclusion**   107
   Reference   110

Index   111

About the Authors

E. Mark Cummings, Ph.D. is a professor and Notre Dame Endowed Chair in psychology at the University of Notre Dame. Guided by the emotional security theory, his work focuses on processes associated with adaptive and maladaptive family functioning and children's and adolescents' development. Dr. Cummings is also interested in relations between family and community contexts and youth development, including pathways to adjustment and well-being in international samples of families exposed to community violence, and relations between political violence, armed conflict, and child development. His current research is also concerned with family- and community-based interventions for families and children.

Christine E. Merrilees, Ph.D. is an assistant professor in the Psychology Department at the State University of New York at Geneseo. Her research uses developmental and social psychological theory with advanced longitudinal methods to assess the impacts of conflict and intergroup divide on youth development. Her work has been published in high-impact journals in developmental, clinical, and social psychology, and her current research focuses on ethnic identity and contact processes that impact well-being and intergroup attitudes and behavior.

Laura K. Taylor, Ph.D. is a lecturer in the School of Psychology with the Centre of Identity and Intergroup Relations at Queen's University, Belfast, Northern Ireland. She has published more than two dozen peer-reviewed articles on her research, which uses a developmental intergroup framework to study risk and resilience processes related to the impact of political violence on children, families, and communities. Her more recent work has focused on constructive outcomes and positive youth development.

Christina F. Mondi, M.A. is a graduate research fellow of the National Science Foundation and a doctoral student in Developmental Psychopathology and Clinical Science at the University of Minnesota. Her research interests are in socio-emotional processes underlying normal development and the development of psychopathology and in school- and family-based early childhood interventions.

Chapter 1
Political Violence, Armed Conflict, and Youth Adjustment: A Worldwide Perspective

Keywords Developmental psychopathology · Armed conflict · Political violence · Social-ecological model · Developmental contexts · Longitudinal research · Translational research

Over one billion youth under the age of 18 are growing up in contexts of political violence and armed conflict worldwide (United Nations, 2009). The conditions and challenges of these young people's lives are diverse, from the wars in the Middle East and Africa, to the crises in Ukraine and Russia, to the lingering tensions of the Troubles of Northern Ireland. While they are often not the focus of public concern, youth are among the most vulnerable victims of political violence and armed conflict. As multiple levels of their social ecologies are disrupted, if not devastated, youth must navigate development without the security of their homes, schools, and communities (Betancourt & Khan, 2008; Boxer et al., 2013; Ladd & Cairns, 1996).

Recent reviews have called attention to the urgency of studying and intervening for youth living in contexts of political violence and armed conflict (Betancourt, Meyers-Ohki, Charrow, & Tol, 2013b; Jordans, Tol, Komproe, & De Jong, 2009; Masten, 2014; Masten & Narayan, 2012). Yet the challenges related to conducting research in these contexts are considerable, and despite an increasing number of published studies in this area in recent years, significant gaps in knowledge remain. There is an urgent need for well-delineated theoretical and methodological approaches that will advance scientific understanding and inform effective translational research and practice.

We concur with Dawes and Cairns' (1998) assertion that we have "counted enough symptoms," and argue that the relationship between exposure to political violence and increased risk of multiple negative outcomes has been well-established in the previous research. We posit that moving forward, there is a critical need for advanced understanding of the following: (a) causal processes that require longitudinal research; (b) the significance of the many levels of youths' social ecologies (e.g., home and community) that are affected by political violence and armed conflict; and (c) cogent implementation of research findings in the development of evidence-based prevention and intervention programs, consistent with the principles of translational research (Cicchetti & Toth, 2006). These recommendations reflect the need for understanding adjustment trajectories from a developmental perspective, including process-oriented tests of treatment effectiveness models (Cummings, Goeke-Morey, Merrilees, Taylor, & Shirlow, 2014; Cummings & Valentino, 2015).

The present book begins by defining the scope of political violence and armed conflict, and by highlighting the urgency of studying youth in these contexts. Next, we introduce the developmental psychopathology as a guiding model for fostering cogent scientific bases for translational work in these contexts (Cummings, Merrilees, Taylor, & Mondi, 2017). We then introduce a four-tier "pyramid" model, grounded in the tenets of developmental psychopathology, for conceptualizing the state of research on political violence, armed conflict, and youth adjustment. This is followed by a review and critique of representative work falling within each respective tier. Finally, we conclude by providing a "road map" of innovative future directions, guided by developmental psychopathology and translational research perspectives, for future research and intervention work in this area.

Whereas the previous reviews have focused on basic or applied research on youth and political violence, the present book systematically demonstrates how basic research should be utilized to inform translational work (Cicchetti & Toth, 2006; Gunnar & Cicchetti, 2009) by reviewing the state of the extant research in this area from a developmental psychopathology perspective (e.g., Cicchetti & Cohen, 2006; Cummings et al., 2017; Cummings & Valentino, 2015). Implicit in this approach are assumptions that: (a) a diverse body of research is essential to optimally inform the development of prevention and intervention programs, and (b) the progression of research in this area can be organized into a conceptually rigorous framework. The extensive, inclusive scope of the review of relevant research and the "road map" grounded in developmental psychopathology and translational research perspectives are among the current book's innovative contributions (e.g., "value added") in relation to previous work (e.g., Attanayake et al., 2009).

Defining Political Violence and Armed Conflict

Our definition of *political violence and armed conflict* refers broadly to contexts involving violent acts with sectarian or group-based (e.g., political, ethnic, religious) motivations. This definition parallels Dubow, Huesmann and Boxer's (2009) designation of *ethnic-political violence* as "violence sanctioned by different influential political and social bodies based on a history of conflict between … groups" (page 114). Notably, we distinguish acts of political violence and armed conflict from other forms of interpersonal violence that lack group-based motivations (e.g., murder, domestic abuse), though political violence and armed conflict may affect these forms of violence (e.g., Cummings et al., 2012b). For the sake of brevity, throughout this book we will interchange the use of the terms *political violence, armed conflict*, and *political violence and armed conflict*, but in all cases we are referring to this more general class of violence.

Our examination of armed conflict encompasses a wide range of violent acts, given that many youth suffer from acts that do not neatly fall within the realms of formal interstate warfare (Cairns, 1996). In the twenty-first century, armed conflict is "more fluid and less easily defined" than in the past (United Nations, 2009). Acts of violence against civilians are increasingly one-sided, fragmented, and perpetrated by non-state actors (e.g., paramilitary, terrorist, or guerilla groups; Stockholm International Peace Research Institute, 2009). Moreover, a wide range of intergroup acts violate human rights, including, but not limited to, acts of terrorism, torture, genocide, riots, and symbolic or expressive acts of intergroup hostility. Furthermore, our concerns with the effects of political violence on youth extend beyond the signing of peace agreements. The repercussions of political violence rarely end with a cease-fire; that is, tension and hostility often linger and continue to affect youth for months and even years after formal conflict has ended (Betancourt, Agnew-Blais, Gilman, Williams, & Ellis, 2010; Betancourt, McBain, Newnham, & Brennan, 2014).

The Urgency of the Study of Youth

Compared to adults, youth affected by political violence and armed conflict have historically received minimal sustained attention by the scientific and public policy communities. Nonetheless, they constitute large proportions of the affected populations. Worldwide, youth are increasingly being recruited as actors in violent conflicts and targeted as victims (Betancourt et al., 2013a). Given the magnitude of this problem, greater knowledge of the specific effects of armed conflict on youth and families is an urgent concern.

Exposure to armed conflict during childhood, compared to exposure later in life, has the potential to be especially detrimental. Young children may have an increased sensitivity to conflict, as early childhood exposure may initiate negative long-term developmental trajectories (see Cummings, George, McCoy & Davies, 2012a; Davies, Sturge-Apple, Boscoe, & Cummings, 2014), including in contexts of political violence (Cummings et al., 2013; Merrilees et al., 2013; Taylor, Merrilees, Goeke-Morey, Shirlow, & Cummings, 2016). During and after periods of active conflict, youth are often exposed to multiple risk factors, including acts of violence, bodily danger, poverty, displacement from their homes and communities, and disruptions of their attachment relationships and educational experiences. These experiences may well exert lasting negative effects on multiple domains of functioning (e.g., cognitive, socio-emotional) that are still developing and emerging throughout childhood (Betancourt, Newnham, McBain, & Brennan, 2013c; Shaw, 2003).

The study of youth in these contexts is also urgent given that they will grow up to become parents, community members, leaders, or combatants, potentially contributing to the intergenerational transmission of conflict and violence. For adolescents, these future roles are quickly approaching. If traumatized youth are not given opportunities to adequately process their experiences, or to engage in peacebuilding efforts (Cummings, Taylor, & Merrilees, 2012c), there is greater risk they will be victimized by or involved in later violent conflicts. Thus, given the unfortunate fact that political violence commonly re-occurs or persists (Darby, 2006), youth represent a critical target for lasting peacebuilding.

Despite the aforementioned risk factors, research indicates that some youth demonstrate remarkable potential for resilience in the face of armed conflict (Barber, 2013; Masten, 2011; 2014). Although resilience processes are important, resilience remains a complex and challenging construct to define and evaluate (Cummings & Valentino, 2015; Luthar, Cicchetti, & Becker, 2000; Ungar, 2015). The individual-, family-, and community-level processes impacted by political violence are complex. Thus, resilience among youth in contexts of political violence requires much future investigation (Masten & Narayan, 2012). Moreover, although resilience merits careful consideration, it is also vital to recognize the great threats that these contexts pose to the well-being of many youth (Betancourt & Khan, 2008). Thus, a goal of this book is to affirm the urgency of developing and disseminating adequately supported prevention and intervention programs that will help youth adaptively process their traumatic experiences, avoid the development of psychopathology, and use their individual, family, and community strengths to grow from their experiences, allowing them to participate constructively in the rebuilding of their communities (Betancourt et al., 2013a; Cummings et al., 2012c; Jordans, Tol, Komproe, & de Jong, 2009).

References

Attanayake, V., McKay, R., Joffres, M., Singh, S., Burkle, F., & Mills, E. (2009). Prevalence of mental disorders among children exposed to war: A systematic review of 7,920 children. *Medicine, Conflict and Survival, 25*(1), 4–19. doi:10.1080/13623690802568913.
Barber, B. K. (2013). Annual research review: The experience of youth with political conflict—challenging notions of resilience and encouraging research refinement. *Journal of Clinical Child Psychology & Psychiatry, 54*(4), 461–473. doi:10.1111/jcpp.12056.
Betancourt, T. S., & Khan, K. T. (2008). The mental health of children affected by armed conflict: Protective processes and pathways to resilience. *International Review of Psychiatry, 20*(3), 317–328. doi:10.1080/09540260802090363.
Betancourt, T. S., Agnew-Blais, J., Gilman, S. E., Williams, D. R., & Ellis, B. H. (2010). Past horrors, present struggles: The role of stigma in the association between war experiences and psychosocial adjustment among former child soldiers in Sierra Leone. *Social Science and Medicine, 70*(1), 17–26. doi:10.1016/j.socscimed.2009.09.038.
Betancourt, T. S., Borisova, I., Williams, T. P., Meyers-Ohki, S. E., Rubin-Smith, J. E., Annan, J., et al. (2013a). Research review: Psychosocial adjustment and mental health in former child soldiers—A systematic review of the literature and recommendations for future research. *Journal of Child Psychology and Psychiatry, 54*(1), 17–36. doi:10.1111/j.1469-7610.2012.02620.x.

Betancourt, T. S., Meyers-Ohki, S. E., Charrow, A. P., & Tol, W. A. (2013b). Interventions for children affected by war: an ecological perspective on psychosocial support and mental health care. *Harvard Review of Psychiatry, 21*(2), 70–91. doi:10.1097/HRP.0b013e318283bf8f.

Betancourt, T. S., Newnham, E. A., McBain, R., & Brennan, R. T. (2013c). Post-traumatic stress symptoms among former child soldiers in Sierra Leone: follow-up study. *British Journal of Psychiatry, 203*(1), 196–202. doi:10.1192/bjp.bp.112.113514.

Betancourt, T. S., McBain, R., Newnham, E. A., & Brennan, R. T. (2014). Context matters: Community characteristics and mental health among war-affected youth in Sierra Leone. *Journal of Child Psychology and Psychiatry, 55*(3), 217–226. doi:10.1111/jccp.12131.

Boxer, P., Huesmann, L. R., Dubow, E. F., Landau, S. F., Gvirsman, S. D., Shikaki, K., et al. (2013). Exposure to violence across the social ecosystem and the development of aggression: A test of ecological theory in the Israeli-Palestinian conflict. *Child Development, 84*(1), 163–177. doi:10.1111/j.1467-8624.2012.01848.x.

Cairns, E. (1996). *Children and political violence*. Hoboken, NJ: Wiley-Blackwell.

Cicchetti, D., & Toth, S. L. (2006). Building bridges and crossing them: Translational research in developmental psychopathology. *Development and Psychopathology, 18*(3), 619–622. doi:10.1017/S0954579406060317.

Cummings, E. M., & Valentino, K. V. (2015). Development Psychopathology. In W. F. Overton & P. C. M. Molenaar (Eds.), *Theory and Method*. Volume 1 of the *Book of child psychology and developmental science*. (7th ed.). (pp. 566–606). Editor-in-Chief: Richard M. Lerner. Hoboken, NJ: Wiley.

Cummings, E. M., George, M. R. W., McCoy, K. P., & Davies, P. T. (2012a). Interparental conflict in kindergarten and adolescent adjustment: Prospective investigation of emotional security as an explanatory mechanism. *Child Development, 83*(5), 1703–1715. doi:10.1111/j.1467-8624.2012.01807.x.

Cummings, E. M., Merrilees, C. E., Schermerhorn, A. C., Goeke-Morey, M. C., Shirlow, P., & Cairns, E. (2012b). Political violence and child adjustment: Longitudinal tests of sectarian antisocial behavior, family conflict and insecurity as explanatory pathways. *Child Development, 83*(2), 461–468. doi:10.1111/j.1467-8624.2011.01720.x.

Cummings, E. M., Taylor, L. K., & Merrilees, C. E. (2012c). A social ecological perspective on risk and resilience for children and political violence: Implications for restoring civil societies. In K. J. Jonas & T. A. Morton (Eds.), *Restoring civil societies: The psychology of intervention and engagement following crisis* (pp. 78–99). Wiley Blackwell: SPSSI series on Social Issues and Interventions.

Cummings, E. M., Taylor, L. K., Merrilees, C. E., Goeke-Morey, M. C., Shirlow, P., & Cairns, E. (2013). Relations between political violence and child adjustment: A four-wave test of the role of emotional insecurity about community. *Developmental Psychology, 49*(12), 2212–2224. doi:10.1037/a0032309.

Cummings, E. M., Goeke-Morey, M. C., Merrilees, C. E., Taylor, L. K., & Shirlow, P. (2014). A social-ecological, process-oriented perspective on political violence and child development. *Child Development Perspectives, 8*(2), 82–89. doi:10.1111/cdep.12067.

Cummings, E., M., Merrilees, C. E., Taylor, L. K., & Mondi, C. F. (2017). Developmental and Social-Ecological Perspectives on Children, Political Violence, and Armed Conflict. *Development and Psychopathology, 29*(1), 1–10. doi:10.1017/S0954579416001061.

Darby, J. (2006). *Violence and reconstruction*. Notre Dame, IN: University of Notre Dame Press.

Davies, P. T., Sturge-Apple, M., Boscoe, S. M., & Cummings, E. M. (2014). The legacy of early insecurity histories in shaping adolescent adaptation to interparental conflict. *Child Development, 85*(1), 338–352. doi:10.1111/cdev.12119.

Dawes, A., & Cairns, E. (1998). The Machel study: Dilemmas of cultural sensitivity and universal rights of children. *Peace and Conflict: Journal of Peace Psychology, 4*(4), 335–348. doi:10.1207/s15327949pac0404_3.

Dubow, E. F., Huesmann, L. R., & Boxer, P. (2009). A social-cognitive-ecological framework for understanding the impact of exposure to persistent ethnic-political violence on children's psychosocial adjustment. *Clinical Child and Family Psychology Review, 12*(2), 113–126. doi:10.1007/s10567-009-0050-7.

Gunnar, M. R., & Cicchetti, D. (2009). Meeting the challenge of translational research in child psychology. In M. R. Gunnar & D. Cicchetti (Eds.), *Meeting the Challenge of Translational Research in Child Psychology: Minnesota Symposia on Child Psychology* (Vol. 35, pp. 1–27). New York: Wiley.

Jordans, M. J. D., Tol, W. A., Komproe, I. H., & de Jong, J. V. T. M. (2009). Systematic review of evidence and treatment approaches: Psychosocial and mental health care for children in war. *Child and Adolescent Mental Health, 14*(1), 2–14. doi:10.1111/j.1475-3588.2008.00515.x.

Ladd, G. W., & Cairns, E. (1996). Children: Ethnic and political violence. *Child Development, 67* (1), 14–18. doi:10.1111/j.1467-8624.1996.tb01715.x.

Luthar, S. S., Cicchetti, D., & Becker, B. (2000). The construct of resilience: A critical evaluation and guidelines for future work. *Child Development, 71*(3), 543–562. doi:10.1111/1467-8624. 00164.

Masten, A. S. (2011). Resilience in children threatened by extreme adversity: Frameworks for research, practice, and translational synergy. *Development and Psychopathology, 23*(2), 493–506. doi:10.1017/S0954579411000198.

Masten, A. S. (2014). Global perspectives on resilience in children and youth. *Child Development, 85*(1), 6–20. doi:10.1111/cdev.12205.

Masten, A., & Narayan, A. J. (2012). Child development in the context of disaster, war, and terrorism: Pathways of risk and resilience. *Annual Review of Psychology, 63,* 227–257. doi:10. 1146/annurev-psych-120710-100356.

Merrilees, C. E., Cairns, E., Taylor, L. K., Goeke-Morey, M. C., Shirlow, P., & Cummings, E. M. (2013). Social identity and youth aggressive and delinquent behaviors in a context of political violence. *Political Psychology, 34*(5), 695–711. doi:10.1111/pops.12030.

Shaw, J. A. (2003). Children exposed to war/terrorism. *Clinical Child and Family Psychology Review, 6*(4), 237–246. doi:10.1023/B:CCFP.0000006291.10180.bd.

Stockholm International Peace Research Institute. (2009). *Sipri yearbook 2009: Armaments, disarmament, and international security.* Oxford: Oxford University Press.

Taylor, L. K., Merrilees, C. E., Goeke-Morey, M. C., Shirlow, P., & Cummings, E. M. (2016). Trajectories of adolescent aggression and family cohesion: The potential to perpetuate or ameliorate political conflict. *Journal of Clinical Child and Adolescent Psychology, 45*(2), 114–28. doi:10.1080/15374416.2014.945213.

Ungar, M. (2015). Practitioner review: Diagnosing childhood resilience—a systemic approach to the diagnosis of adaptation in adverse social and physical ecologies. *Journal of Child Psychology and Psychiatry, 56*(1), 4–17. doi:10.1111/jcpp.12306.

United Nations Children Fund. (2009). *Machel study 10-year strategic review: Children and conflict in a changing world.* New York: Office of the Special Representative of the Secretary-General for Children and Armed Conflict.

Chapter 2
Developmental Psychopathology as a Guiding Model

Keywords Developmental psychopathology · Political violence · Armed conflict · Translational research · Mediators · Moderators · Social-ecological model

As a guiding model for process-oriented and translational research (Cummings & Valentino, 2015), we posit that the tenets of developmental psychopathology can facilitate significant advancements in the study of youth affected by political violence and armed conflict (Cummings et al., 2017). Developmental psychopathology has the overarching goal of integrating the developmental and clinical sciences to study explanatory models of normal and abnormal development, including understanding positive trajectories, resilience, and to inform approaches to prevention and treatment (Cummings, Davies, & Campbell, 2000). A central concern is articulating the dynamic developmental processes that underlie negative outcomes, including but not limited to clinical psychopathology, as well as positive or resilient outcomes. Fundamental assumptions include the following: (a) psychopathology is not a disease (that is, a pathogenic entity within the individual) but rather reflects maladaptive processes of functioning; and (b) normal and abnormal processes develop over time, and are subject to change course; and (c) youth functioning must be understood in relation to developmental processes and other contextual elements (Cicchetti, 2006; Cicchetti & Cohen, 1995). That is, development is an ongoing interplay between an active, always changing child, and an active, changing context.

The developmental psychopathology perspective outlines how interplaying influences across multiple contexts (e.g., biological, social, and cultural) contribute to positive or negative development across the lifespan. From this perspective, the identification of a problem and its correlates—for example, the number of youth affected by political violence and armed conflict who develop psychological symptoms—only establishes that there is a problem that needs to be addressed, not *why*, *how*, *when*, and *for whom* the problem develops, nor how the problem should be addressed. Emphasis is thus placed on uncovering the *processes* underlying particular developmental outcomes, with the ultimate goal of translating this knowledge into interventions to promote healthier outcomes. Emphasis is also

E.M. Cummings et al., *Political Violence, Armed Conflict, and Youth Adjustment*,
DOI 10.1007/978-3-319-51583-0_2

placed on identifying contextual issues and individual differences that may help identify for whom or under what conditions prevention or intervention will be most effective. The latter goals may be accomplished in contexts of political violence by conducting research that is guided by developmental theory, that employs multiple methods and levels of analysis, and that uses longitudinal research designs (e.g., Boxer et al., 2013; Cummings, Goeke-Morey, Merrilees, Taylor, & Shirlow, 2014; Cummings et al., 2013; Cummings, Merrilees, Taylor, Goeke-Morey, & Shirlow, 2017; Merrilees, Taylor, Goeke-Morey, Shirlow, & Cummings, 2014; Dubow et al., 2012).

Finally, consistent with Bronfenbrenner's (1977, 1979) social-ecological model and the developmental psychopathology perspective, another central emphasis necessary for substantial scientific advances is on relations between youth and the many contexts in which they develop. Thus, another direction emphasized in this book is the evaluation of the influence of risk and protective processes at multiple social-ecological levels on youth, including the family, school, and community (Elbedour, ten Bensel, & Bastien, 1993). This focus also informs our analysis of factors that may influence the effectiveness of interventions for youth.

Fostering Cogent Scientific Bases for Prevention and Intervention: Translational Research

Basic research conducted under the guiding model of developmental psy-chopathology is optimally positioned to serve as a foundation for subsequent translational research. The goal of translational research is to use basic research to inform prevention and intervention efforts and, consequently, improve develop-mental outcomes (Cummings & Valentino, 2015). The National Institutes of Mental Health have advocated for increased translational research, as reflected in a road map (National Advisory Mental Health Council, 2000) that prioritizes research that capitalizes on basic research findings in the prevention and treatment of disease (Zerhouni, 2003). From this perspective, prevention and intervention programs should not be constructed ad hoc, or merely reflect disciplinary fiat regarding approach. Rather, they should have firm and systematic bases in empirical work. This conceptualization of research with the purpose of improving public health is described in the medical field as reflecting the transition of research findings from "bench to bedside" (Insel, 2005). The "bench to bedside" direction emphasizes the application of knowledge gained from basic research to the development and evaluation of prevention or intervention approaches (Insel, 2009). Basic research that advances understanding of the causal processes underlying both adjustment and maladjustment is regarded as a particularly optimal foundation for translational work (Cicchetti & Toth, 2006).

There is also increasing emphasis on achieving a goal of bidirectional relations between basic research and research in clinical settings—that is, "bedside to bench." Hypotheses about mediating and moderating developmental processes can be tested during clinical evaluations of prevention or intervention programs in appropriate and scientifically valuable ways, thereby also contributing to knowledge of the nature and course of adjustment and maladjustment (Cicchetti & Toth, 2006). Interventions that generate data on causal processes and moderators may help to further refine program content and to target services to appropriate populations.

References

Boxer, P., Huesmann, L. R., Dubow, E. F., Landau, S. F., Gvirsman, S. D., Shikaki, K., et al. (2013). Exposure to violence across the social ecosystem and the development of aggression: A test of ecological theory in the Israeli-Palestinian conflict. *Child Development, 84*(1), 163–177. doi:10.1111/j.1467-8624.2012.01848.x.

Bronfenbrenner, U. (1977). Toward an experimental ecology of human development. *American Psychologist, 32*(7), 513–541. doi:10.1037/0003-066X.32.7.513.

Bronfenbrenner, U. (1979). *The ecology of human development: Experiments by nature and design*. Cambridge, MA: Harvard University Press.

Cicchetti, D. (2006). Development and psychopathology. In D. Cicchetti & D. J. Cohen (Eds.), *Developmental psychopathology : Vol. 1. Theory and methods* (pp. 1–23). New York: Wiley.

Cicchetti, D., & Cohen, D. J. (1995). Perspectives on developmental psychopathology. In D. Cicchetti & D. J. Cohen (Eds.), *Developmental psychopathology : Vol. 1. Theory and methods* (pp. 3–20). New York: Wiley.

Cicchetti, D., & Toth, S. L. (2006). Building bridges and crossing them: Translational research in developmental psychopathology. *Development and Psychopathology, 18*(3), 619–622. doi:10.1017/S0954579406060317.

Cummings, E. M., Davies, P. T., & Campbell, S. B. (2000). *Developmental psychopathology and family process: Theory, research, and clinical implications*. New York: Guilford Press.

Cummings, E. M., Merrilees, C. E., Taylor, L. K., Shirlow, P., Goeke-Morey, M. C., & Cairns, E. (2013). Longitudinal relations between sectarian and nonsectarian community violence and child adjustment in Northern Ireland. *Development and Psychopathology, 25*(3), 615–627. doi:10.1017/S0954579413000059.

Cummings, E. M., Goeke-Morey, M. C., Merrilees, C. E., Taylor, L. K., & Shirlow, P. (2014). A social-ecological, process-oriented perspective on political violence and child development. *Child Development Perspectives, 8*(2), 82–89. doi:10.1111/cdep.12067.

Cummings, E. M., & Valentino, K. V. (2015). Development Psychopathology. In W. F. Overton & P. C. M. Molenaar (Eds.), *Theory and method*. Volume 1 of *the Handbook* of *child psychology and developmental science*. (7th ed., pp. 566–606). Editor-in-Chief: Richard M. Lerner. Hoboken, NJ: Wiley.

Cummings, E. M., Merrilees, C. E., Taylor, L. K., & Mondi, C. F. (2017). Developmental and social-ecological perspectives on children, political violence, and armed conflict. *Development and Psychopathology, 29*(1), 1–10. doi:10.1017/S0954579416001061.

Cummings, E. M., Merrilees, C. E., Taylor, L. K., Goeke-Morey, M. C., & Shirlow, P. (2017). Emotional insecurity about the community: A dynamic, within-person mediator of child adjustment in contexts of political violence. *Development and Psychopathology, 29*(1), 27–36. doi:10.1017/S0954579416001097.

Dubow, E. F., Huesmann, L. R., Boxer, P., Landau, S., Dvir, S., Shikaki, K., et al. (2012). Exposure to political conflict and violence and posttraumatic stress in middle east youth: Protective factors. *Journal of Clinical Child and Adolescent Psychology, 41*(4), 402–416. doi:10.1080/15374416.2012.684274.

Elbedour, S., ten Bensel, R., & Bastien, D. T. (1993). Ecological integrated model of children of war: Individual and social psychology. *Child Abuse and Neglect, 17*(6), 805–819.

Insel, T. R. (2005). Developmental psychobiology for public health: A bridge for translational research. *Developmental Psychobiology, 47*(3), 209–216. doi:10.1002/dev.20089.

Insel, T. R. (2009). Translating scientific opportunity into public health impact: A strategic plan for research on mental illness. *Archives of General Psychiatry, 66*(2), 128–133. doi:10.1001/archgenpsychiatry.2008.540.

Merrilees, C. E., Taylor, L. K., Goeke-Morey, M. C., Shirlow, P., & Cummings, E. M. (2014). Youth in contexts of political violence: A developmental approach to the study of youth identity and emotional security in their communities. *Peace and Conflict: Journal of Peace Psychology, 20*(1), 26–39. doi:10.1080/10781910903088932.

National Advisory Mental Health Council. (2000). *Translating behavioral science into action: Report of the national advisory mental health council's behavioral science workgroup* (no. 00-4699). Bethesda, MD: National Institutes of Mental Health.

Zerhouni, E. (2003). The NIH roadmap. *Science, 302*(5642), 63–72. doi:10.1126/science.1091867.

Chapter 3
A Framework: Review of Research from a Developmental Psychopathology Perspective

Keywords Political violence · Armed conflict · Social-ecological model · Longitudinal designs · Translational research

At this point, we draw from the tenets of developmental psychopathology to analyze the themes and patterns of previous research on youth, political violence, and armed conflict. Implicit in this approach are the assumptions that a diverse body of basic empirical research is essential to adequately inform the development of effective prevention and intervention programs and that the progression of this research can be organized into a conceptually rigorous framework that: (a) establishes the existence of risk for maladjustment; (b) begins to articulate processes related to risk and protection via cross-sectional research; (c) investigates the processes underlying risk and protection via longitudinal research; and (d) translates basic research findings into intervention development, including the evaluation of program efficacy and the process-oriented study of why programs do or do not work.

In this regard, we conceptualize the published research in this area in terms of a *four-tiered pyramid* that "builds up" to a goal of targeted prevention and intervention programs for affected youth (see Fig. 3.1). The four tiers of research which we identify and will review in this book are: (a) studies documenting youth outcomes in contexts of political violence and armed conflict, including empirical support for the effects of level of exposure on youth outcomes and demographic moderators of outcomes (*Tier 1*, exemplified in Table 4.1); (b) studies exploring mediators, process-oriented moderators, and social-ecological contexts that are salient to youth outcomes, using *primarily cross-sectional designs* (*Tier 2*, exemplified in Table 5.1); (c) studies that empirically test the underlying mechanisms and critical social-ecological contexts by which youth arrive at particular outcomes, using *primarily longitudinal designs* (*Tier 3*, exemplified in Table 6.1); and (d) studies that utilize Tier 3 research findings to develop and evaluate prevention and intervention programs (Tier 4).

Each tier of this pyramid contributes critically to the foundation for subsequent tiers, reflecting progressively greater demands for theoretical and methodological rigor. For example, Tier 1 research documenting heightened rates of psychological

© Springer International Publishing AG 2017
E.M. Cummings et al., *Political Violence, Armed Conflict, and Youth Adjustment*,
DOI 10.1007/978-3-319-51583-0_3

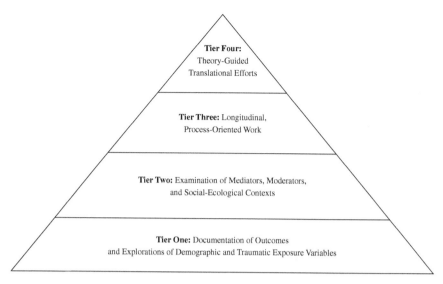

Fig. 3.1 A framework for research on children, political violence, and armed conflict: a developmental psychopathology perspective

problems among youth affected by political violence serves as an important impetus for the investment of time and resources into exploration of the mediators, moderators, and social-ecological contexts that contribute to such outcomes (Tiers 2 and 3). Likewise, prevention and intervention programs (Tier 4) will be best positioned to meaningfully enhance youth well-being when they systematically target critical developmental mechanisms and social-ecological contexts, as identified by methodologically rigorous basic research (Tier 3).

Thus, we envision that researchers working at the top of the pyramid (Tier 4) would ideally focus on developing and evaluating prevention and intervention programs that build on the findings of the basic research studies reflected in lower tiers, especially Tier 3, when they are available. Despite an increasing number of published studies on such programs, there have been varying levels of rigor and few studies qualified for this tier (see Table 7.1 for examples of studies that incorporate many, but not all elements of the translational approach). Although much of the research shown in Table 7.1 work is marked by innovation and merit, the process of translating empirical developmental and clinical research into the design and delivery of prevention and intervention programs has been limited.

It is important to acknowledge that, while the ultimate goal of translational research is to effectively infuse basic research into novel and effective intervention efforts, the process of moving between basic and translational work may be iterative, with multiple strategies underway and contributing to knowledge at the same time (Gunnar & Cicchetti, 2009). Moving information along a path from scientific discovery to developing and testing new intervention approaches may progress in multiple ways from any point in the pyramid we have outlined to the next, as gaps in knowledge are filled in. However, the cost of research in terms of time and resources is likely to increase substantially as one goes up the pyramid. In some cases, given the urgency of the problems faced by youth living in contexts of political violence, it may be necessary to test theories of change or protection through intervention and evaluation research, rather than waiting until the whole pyramid foundation is completed. Robust evaluation of programs' effects is especially essential in these cases. It is also critical in these cases that intervention efforts draw from existing literature at lower tiers that most closely relate to the experiences of youth in a given context. For example, if research has not been completed in a giving context, researchers can draw from existing theory and research for youth exposed to community violence in the USA. Yet, without a solid foundation of research and theories about processes of change or protection (as best established by Tier 3 research), such intervention efforts may be risky, costly, and have limited prospects for success or may even exert unintentional negative consequences on youth. We therefore believe that, in the long term, investing in the development of a solid foundation of Tiers 1–3 research greatly increases the likelihood of substantive payoffs in the form of more effective, cost-effective programs at the Tier 4 level.

In this book, we will use the four-tiered pyramid, based on the tenets of developmental psychopathology, to consider how current research advances our understanding of youth adjustment and maladjustment in contexts of political violence. We will then outline multiple practical, theoretical, and methodological strategies to facilitate strategic movement up the pyramid, toward advances in knowledge, prevention, and intervention in this area.

Methodology: Search Strategy for Identifying Tier 1–3 Studies

We conducted a large-scale literature review on youth adjustment in contexts of political violence and armed conflict, comprehensively sampling Tiers 1–3 research. The literature review for Tier 4 was conducted in a supplemental search and is described below. Our review was comprehensive; however, our goal in the current book is to convey the details of representative studies from each tier of our conceptual pyramid. The three tables 4.1, 5.1, and 6.1 bring to the forefront, with rich levels of detail, the key characteristics of the vibrant literature on political violence, armed conflict, and youth adjustment.

The initial review was conducted using PsycINFO and Web of Science between spring 2012 and summer 2013, followed by additional searches for new publications conducted in autumn 2014 and summer 2015. Search terms were refined across multiple rounds of online searching and in consultation with a psychology librarian. Multiple synonyms for political violence and armed conflict (e.g., political conflict, ethnic violence/conflict, war), youth (e.g., children, adolescents),

internalizing and externalizing behaviors and symptoms (e.g., aggression, delinquency, depression, post-traumatic stress disorder), and notably, positive behaviors
and attitudes (e.g., participation, empathy, forgiveness, prejudice) were employed.
Early search results were cross-checked with the reference lists of key and highly
cited articles on youth, political violence, and armed conflict. Forward and back-
ward searches were also conducted on key and highly cited articles. Accordingly,
given the breadth of studies identified by our search criteria, and the common
inclusion of multiple youth outcomes in these studies, the representation of research
on multiple youth outcomes was extensive. In all, a total of 795 studies were
identified.

After initial collection efforts, excluded from further examination were studies
that: (a) were not published in peer-reviewed journals or academic books, including
dissertations; (b) were not published in English; (c) were not primarily focused on
youth populations under the age of 25 (e.g., studies in which adult participants
living as refugees or immigrants in new host countries recalled their childhood
experiences with political violence), reflecting this book's focus on youth who may
currently benefit from prevention or intervention efforts; (d) were published before
1990; or (e) employed solely qualitative methods, or made assumptions about, but
did not empirically measure, whether participants had been exposed to acts of
political violence. These criteria may have excluded some high-quality studies that
were not published in English or excellent qualitative studies; however, the aim of
this book was not to be exhaustive in its coverage of previous work, but to reflect
the state of the art at each tier of the pyramid.

Of the total sample of 795 articles that were identified, approximately one-third
qualified for initial review in the present book. Critically, this book will discuss the
broader set of studies found in the review process, while a subset of those studies
will be presented in the first three tables as illustrative exemplars of the types of
studies that are encompassed by each respective tier of the pyramid. As readers will
see, the studies falling within each tier are diverse in terms of their designs and
geographies, but reflect overarching conceptual and methodological similarities that
distinguish them from studies in other tiers (see Fig. 3.1). Research at each tier level
provides a critical empirical foundation upon which studies and interventions in
subsequent tiers can be built. Upon examination of the sampling of studies presented in the first three tables, it is evident that variables and questions are explored
with increasing complexity and rigor as one moves up the pyramid. Relatedly,
studies in lower tiers of the pyramid are ideally suited for addressing foundational
questions (e.g., exposure effects, impact on multiple psychological and health
symptoms) because they may be more amenable to collection of large sample sizes
and less expensive in terms of funding, time, and resources.

The first three tables (reflecting Tiers 1–3, respectively) present diverse sampling
of these studies representing work from around the globe. In the interest of space,
20 studies are presented per table. When selecting studies to present in the tables,
several considerations were made. Our first consideration was to represent research
from multiple geographic regions affected by political violence and armed conflict,
including Africa, Asia, and Europe. A second related consideration was to present

studies examining distinct political conflicts from each of these regions. A third consideration was to compile a body of studies that, taken together, examined multiple independent and dependent variables. A fourth consideration was to include studies examining a wide age range of youth. Finally, whenever possible, we endeavored to include studies from diverse research groups. With that being said, given that less work has been done at the Tier 3 versus Tiers 1 or 2 levels, several research groups are represented multiple times in Table 6.1. In the context of all the latter considerations, studies with large sample sizes, strong sampling procedures, complex statistical analyses, and other evidence of methodological rigor and sophistication were favored for inclusion (see Barenbaum, Ruchkin, & Schwab-Stone, 2004).

The added value of presenting detailed information on a substantial sampling of studies at each tier is that it provides a ready reference for the characteristics and qualities of specific studies conducted throughout the world on political violence, armed conflict, and youth, including research designs, ages of participants, assessments, timing of the studies in relation to political violence or armed conflict, and key findings. Thus, an accessible book is provided with regard to the status and characteristics of specific research studies drawn from throughout the world, including a quick overview of key studies at each level of analysis reflecting the worldwide literature. Notably, focus on only the highest quality, process-oriented longitudinal studies ignores a vast literature of important studies and also yields a limited perspective on the work done toward understanding mediators and moderators of youth outcomes worldwide, since studies are limited to a small number of research laboratories in a limited number of areas of study (see Table 6.1). By contrast, a wider, richer consideration of hypothesis generation and analysis emerges from an examination of Tier 1 and 2 studies, albeit less rigorously tested given the reliance on cross-sectional research designs. Studies reflecting Tiers 1 and 2 provide vast amounts of valuable and insightful information, reflecting high-quality work selected from a much larger literature on this topic (i.e., $N = 795$ studies). The goal of this book was to provide a useful book of the state of the art, while at the same time providing directions toward new advances in the future.

References

Barenbaum, J., Ruchkin, V., & Schwab-Stone, M. (2004). The psychosocial aspects of children exposed to war: Practice and policy initiatives. *Journal of Child Psychology and Psychiatry, 45* (1), 41–62. doi:10.1046/j.0021-9630.2003.00304.x.

Gunnar, M. R., & Cicchetti, D. (2009). Meeting the challenge of translational research in child psychology. In M. R. Gunnar & D. Cicchetti (Eds.), *Meeting the challenge of translational research in child psychology: Minnesota symposia on child psychology* (Vol. 35, pp. 1–27). New York: Wiley.

Chapter 4
Tier 1 Studies: Documenting the Impact on Youth

Keywords Political violence · Armed conflict · Youth adjustment · Posttraumatic stress disorder · Cross-sectional studies · Risk · Resilience · Violence exposure · Externalizing problems

The population at hand—youth affected by political violence—went largely unstudied until the twentieth century. During this era, three major factors—the rise of the social sciences, increasing interest in child development, and the eruption of numerous wars across the globe—converged to motivate research on the psychological effects of childhood exposure to political violence and armed conflict. A growing body of research in this area has emerged over the past century. In the following section, we will highlight the findings of this historic body of work, discuss our conceptualization of Tier 1 studies, and review the current literature on this topic.

Historic Research

Florence Young (1947) summarized the concerns of many psychologists and laypeople of the time, writing: "The postwar era will be guided by those who were children...during World War II. If the war has caused large numbers of them to have deep-seated maladjustments, the future will be correspondingly jeopardized" (p. 500). It was under these premises that twentieth-century researchers and clinicians set out to document the psychological outcomes of war-exposed youth.

Interestingly, several early research reviews concluded that youth did not appear to be as psychologically damaged by wartime experiences as had been initially anticipated (e.g., Despert, 1944). Several studies reported that most youths' psychological problems significantly decreased in the months and years following war exposure (e.g., Burt, 1940). Among those who did continue to demonstrate psychological problems, several common threads were identified—for example, lower average intelligence (e.g., John, 1941), dysfunctional family dynamics (e.g., Bodman & Dunsdon, 1941), and direct exposure to bombing attacks (e.g., Bodman, 1941).

© Springer International Publishing AG 2017

E.M. Cummings et al., *Political Violence, Armed Conflict, and Youth Adjustment*,
DOI 10.1007/978-3-319-51583-0_4

Some researchers also suggested that haphazard evacuations and disruptions of attachment relationships (e.g., separation from parents) were actually more psychologically distressing experiences for youth than exposure to military events (e.g., Alcock, 1941; Burbury, 1941; Burt, 1940; Freud & Burlingham, 1943).

These early studies provided important information about the psychological effects of exposure to political violence on youth. They drew public and scientific attention to the millions of youth caught up in the wars of their times, while also challenging the prevailing notion that all of them were destined for serious maladjustment. Nonetheless, it is critical to acknowledge the gaps, discrepancies, and methodological problems that are prevalent in this early corpus of work. Early studies frequently reported on youth adjustment based on parental report or general clinical impressions, resulting in vague accounts of psychological symptoms. For example, Bodman (1941) described signs of "strain" among young evacuees, encompassing a wide range of psychological (e.g., "general nervousness, trembling, crying, and aggressive behavior") and psychosomatic symptoms (e.g., "headaches, anorexia, indigestion, enuresis, soiling, pallor, and epistaxis"). Some of these symptoms are consistent with the modern diagnosis of posttraumatic stress disorder (PTSD); however, like many early studies, this study's original two-page report (Bodman, 1941) provided extremely limited information about participants' exact experiences and trajectories. The absence of detailed information and standardized measurement makes it difficult to evaluate discrepancies that emerged between studies in this era—for example, conflicting findings about whether younger or older children tended to fare better psychologically postwar.

During the mid-twentieth century, following the end of World War II, research on the effects of political violence and armed conflict on children became fewer and farther between. Following the 1967 Arab Israeli War, Ziv and Israel (1973) reported no differences in manifest anxiety symptoms between children living in bombarded versus non-bombarded Israeli settlements. In a similar vein, Ziv, Kruglanski, and Shulman (1974) compared the psychological reactions of Israeli children who lived in shelled versus non-shelled settlements. They reported that children living in shelled settlements exhibited more patriotism, covert aggression, and appreciation for courage than those who did not live in shelled settlements— possibly reflecting active attempts to cope with ongoing stress. Other researchers began to explore questions about youths' emerging ideologies and political socialization to international conflict (e.g., Tolley, 1973). In 1982, the journalist Roger Rosenblatt published a *Time* cover story containing interviews with children from five international war zones, which eventually turned into an award-winning book (Rosenblatt, 1983). By the 1980s, more research and media attention were returning to youth living in contexts of political violence and armed conflict.

This historic review brings us to the current literature that covers the spike in global armed conflict after the end of the Cold War. The following section presents our conceptualization of Tier 1 research and reviews' representative studies from this tier.

Recent Studies

Since the end of the Cold War, recent research has introduced new and more rigorous classification and measurement systems for studying youth adjustment in diverse contexts of armed conflict. A primary contribution has been to document the incidence, prevalence, and diverse forms of developmental outcomes experienced by youth with different demographic characteristics and exposure experiences throughout the world. For example, the studies presented in Table 4.1 provide evidence, frequently based on impressive sample sizes and psychometrically sound measurement, for statistically significant links between exposure to political violence and maladjustment across the globe, from Africa (e.g., Darfur, Rwanda, South Africa, and Uganda) to Europe (e.g., Bosnia-Herzegovina, Croatia, and Northern Ireland) and Asia (e.g., Cambodia, Nepal, Lebanon, Palestine, and Israel).

Returning to the previously introduced pyramid framework for conceptualizing the progression of research in this area (Fig. 3.1), the studies presented in Table 4.1 reflect work conduced at the Tier 1 level. By our definition, Tier 1 research documents youth outcomes in contexts of armed conflict, including consideration of the role of demographic (e.g., age and gender) and exposure variables. This tier of research, which demonstrates the impact on youth, constitutes an essential building block for understanding the nature of the challenges facing youth in contexts of political violence. The identification of demographic moderators (e.g., age and gender) may provide important clues as to the nature of relations between political violence and child outcomes. Nonetheless, from a developmental psychopathology perspective, Tier 1 studies, which typically employ cross-sectional designs, make limited progress toward informing understanding about the *dynamic processes* (e.g., dynamic mediators) and modifiable moderators that are related to particular outcomes and that could be mitigated or enhanced to address questions about why particular youth arrive at particular outcomes. Thus, studies at Tier 1 studies thus provide limited foundation for the design and delivery of translational prevention or intervention work.

We identified approximately 125 published studies that fit the Tier 1 criteria. We will now discuss noteworthy findings and patterns from this body of work. Additionally, as discussed in Chapter 4, we employed a number of criteria to select a diverse subset of Tier 1 studies ($N = 20$) to present in detail in Table 4.1.

Youth Outcomes

Several trends are noteworthy in the Tier 1 literature: (a) extensive reporting on psychopathology symptoms, especially posttraumatic stress disorder (PTSD); (b) wide variability in the documented rates and severities of the aforementioned conditions; (c) exploration of the links between demographic variables (e.g., age and gender), traumatic exposure type, and youth adjustment; and (d) burgeoning interest in studying resilience processes among affected youth. At the same time, unresolved questions about the definition, measurement, and scope of resiliency remain.

In all parts of the world, exposure to political violence has been linked to heightened rates of psychological problems (see Table 4.1). PTSD is perhaps the most frequently studied form of psychological maladjustment in youth affected by political violence. In a recent meta-analysis, Attanayake and colleagues (2009) reported that PTSD was the primary outcome of interest of all 17 studies that they reviewed, with an overall pooled prevalence rate of 47%. Other studies have reported that the percentage of sampled youth meeting clinical criteria for PTSD was 75% in Darfur (Morgos, Worden, & Gupta, 2007); 97% in Uganda (Derluyn, Broekart, Schuyten, & De Temmerman, 2004); and 94% in Bosnia-Herzegovina (Goldstein, Wampler, & Wise, 1997). After PTSD, the next most common psychological problems in Attanayake and colleagues' review were depression and anxiety disorders, with pooled prevalence estimates of 43 and 27%, respectively. However, given the limited scope of assessment in survey studies, these rates may be underestimates and multiple other problems may be prevalent.

Reported rates, severities, and durations of psychological symptoms vary widely, and comorbid problems are common (e.g., see Table 4.1). According to Shaw (2003), the prevalence estimates for clinically significant problems among children exposed to war and terrorism range from 10 to 90%, with exposure dose effects identified as the most important predictor of negative adjustment outcomes. Several considerations offer insight into the sources of variability in the patterns of youth outcomes across Tier 1 studies. These factors include (a) sample demographic characteristics (e.g., gender and age), (b) source and intensity of violence exposure and time elapsed between exposure and outcome assessment, and (c) context-specific differences in exposure to political violence.

First, demographic characteristics have been related to individuals' probabilities of developing psychopathology in contexts of political violence and armed conflict (see Fazel, Reed, Panter-Brick, & Stein, 2012). Age and gender are the most commonly studied variables, with significant but, to some extent, conflicting results regarding which ages and gender are associated with highest risk (see Table 4.1). For example, when gender differences are found, particularly in studies focusing on internalizing problems, higher rates of psychological symptoms are typically reported among females than males (e.g., Giacaman, Shannon, Saab, Arya, & Boyce, 2007; Okello, De Schryver, Musisi, Broekaert, & Derluyn, 2014; Smith, Perrin, Yule, Hacam, & Stuvland, 2002). On the other hand, for other problem behaviors, such as aggression, higher rates are reported among males than females (e.g., Al-Krenawai & Graham, 2012). Likewise, some studies have reported higher rates of psychological symptoms among older youth (e.g., Ahmad, von Knorring, & Sundelin-Wahlstein, 2008; Goldstein et al., 1997), whereas others have reported higher rates among younger youth (Schwarzwald, Weisenberg, Waysman, Solomon, & Klingman, 1993), or no significant differences among youth of different genders or ages (e.g., Klasen, Oettingen, Daniels, & Adams, 2010; Lev-Wiesel, Al-Krenawi, & Schwail, 2007). Although age and gender differences may potentially be proxies for other risk factors, such as different rates of exposure to political violence (e.g., Vizek-Vidović, Kuterovac-Jagodić, & Arumbašić, 2000), explanations for these results have varied widely, often relying on conjecture rather than empirical evidence at this level of analysis. Nonetheless, the identification of age and gender as potentially salient moderators aligns with a developmental psychopathology perspective on individual difference variables that may interact to predict different outcomes.

Second, different patterns of findings across youth outcomes may be related to different trauma types and severities, as well as the amount of time elapsed between exposure and assessment (Dimitry, 2011). Typically, the highest rates of developmental and psychological problems are reported among youth exposed to recent (e.g., Sack, Clarke, & Seeley, 1996), highly proximal (e.g., Kasler, Dahan, & Elias, 2008; Ronen, Rahav, & Appel, 2003; Schiff et al., 2006), frequent (e.g., Allwood, Bell-Dolan, & Husain, 2002; Miller, El-Masri, Allodi, & Qouta, 1999), and/or highly intense events (e.g., Goldstein et al., 1997). Problems may be acute or long-lasting (Sagi-Schwartz, 2008) and may emerge anytime from immediately after traumatic exposure, up to many years later. To the latter point, many youth living in contexts of political violence are exposed to ongoing adversity, making it difficult to parse out the effects of specific experiences. Direct exposure to conflict, even at high levels, is unlikely to be the sole predictor of risk for maladjustment.

Third, different patterns of youth outcomes across Tier 1 studies may be explained by cultural differences. For example, although PTSD may be assessed using similar criteria, the implications of symptoms may vary widely across cultural settings. In addition, the manifestation of adjustment and maladjustment may differ across contexts. For example, Palestinian youths' activities in the Intifada may be conceptualized as externalizing problems. However, some would argue that these behaviors are psychologically adaptive and that a Western approach to externalizing should not be applied in this case (Punamäki, 1996). At the same time, cross-cultural comparisons are needed, which can be facilitated by universal measures. Thus, it is thus essential to examine the cultural and conflict-specific contexts of armed conflict when assessing youth adjustment and to identify the similarities and differences of these contexts when comparing findings across studies (Barber, 2013, see Table 4.1). However, studies sometimes provide limited information about the cultures, communities, and conflicts surrounding their samples, making the aforementioned considerations very difficult to accommodate.

Table 4.1 Tier 1

Region and conflict	Reference	Sample	Assessment Timing	Measures	Major Findings
Africa					
Rwanda; Rwandan Genocide	Dyregrov, Gupta, Gjestad, and Mukanoheli (2000)	• 3,030 youth (aged 8–19 years) sampled from unaccompanied centers and schools	• Data collection occurred 13 months after the genocide started	• Exposure to war events • Psychological impact of events • Grief reactions	• Exposure to violence, traumatic loss, and fearing for one's life were positively associated with PTSD symptoms • Participants living in shelters reported the highest levels of exposure to violence, but the lowest levels of PTSD reactions
South Africa; ongoing community conflict and political transition	Stone, Kaminer, and Durrheim (2000)	• 540 youth (*M* age = 15.6 years) sampled from a school with almost exclusively black students and a school with almost exclusively white students	• Data collection occurred 2 years after the African National Congress came to power, 4 years after the repeal of apartheid laws	• Political life events • Stressful life events • Psychological symptoms	• Exposure to political life events was positively associated with psychological symptoms, above and beyond the contributions of other stressful life events • A positive linear relationship emerged between exposure to political life events and distress severity
Uganda; Lord's Resistance Army insurgency	Klasen, Oettingen, Daniels, and Adam (2010)	• 330 former Ugandan child soldiers (*M* age = 14.4 years) attending a special needs school for war-traumatized youth.	• Data collection occurred during a period of ongoing conflict	• Traumatic war experiences • Exposure to domestic and community violence • PTSD • Depression • Behavioral and emotional problems	• Traumatic war experiences and domestic violence exposure were both positively associated with PTSD symptoms, depression symptoms, and behavioral and emotional problems • 33% of participants exhibited PTSD symptoms, 36% exhibited depressive symptoms, and 61% exhibited significant behavioral and emotional problems. • No significant gender differences emerged for PTSD symptoms, depressive symptoms, or behavioral and emotional problems
Uganda; Lord's Resistance Army insurgency	Okello, Onen, and Musisi (2007)	• 153 youth (*M* age = 15.2 years for girls and 15.5 years for boys), including youth who had and had not been abducted (unmatched; *n* = 82 and 71, respectively.)	• Data collection occurred during a period of ongoing conflict	• Exposure to traumatic events • Psychiatric symptoms • Psychological distress	• Over 90% of participants reported direct or indirect exposure to severe trauma • Abducted participants exhibited higher levels of PTSD, depression, generalized anxiety disorder, and psychological distress than non-abducted participants • Non-abducted participants reported higher levels of past suicidality

(continued)

Table 4.1 (continued)

Region and conflict	Reference	Sample	Assessment Timing	Measures	Major Findings
					• Despite high rates of psychiatric disorder, participants exhibited overall good psychosocial adjustment
Uganda; Second Sudanese Civil War	Paardekooper, de Jong and Hermanns (1999)	• Sudanese refugee youth living in Uganda (*n* = 316, *M* age = 9.36 years) and Ugandan youth without experiences of war or flight (*n* = 80, *M* age = 9.42 years.)	• Data were collected in Uganda, while conflict was ongoing in Sudan.	• Traumatic experiences • Daily stressors • Coping • Social support • Psychological symptoms (youth and caregiver report)	• Sudanese participants reported greater exposure to traumatic events, more daily stressors, lower satisfaction with received social support, and greater use of coping strategies than Ugandan participants • Sudanese participants reported higher levels of PTSD, depressive, and behavioral symptoms
Asia					
Cambodia; Cambodian humanitarian crisis	Mollica, Poole, Son, Murray, and Tor (1997)	•182 parent–child dyads (youth aged 12–13 years) living in refugee camps on the Cambodian–Thai border	• Data collection occurred during a period of ongoing conflict	• Youth traumatic life experiences (youth and parent reports) • Youth behavioral and emotional symptoms (youth and parent reports) • Youth physical health (parent report) • Educational, social, and cultural experiences in the camp (youth and parent reports)	• Parents and youth reported high levels of cumulative trauma and behavioral and emotional problems among youth • Significant dose-effect relationships emerged between cumulative trauma and all parent-reported symptom scales • Significant dose-effect relationships emerged between cumulative trauma and youth-reported anxiety, depressive, and attention problems • No significant dose-effect relationships emerged between cumulative trauma, social functioning, or physical health status

(continued)

Table 4.1 (continued)

Region and conflict	Reference	Sample	Assessment Timing	Measures	Major Findings
Israel and disputed districts; Israeli–Palestinian Conflict	Solomon and Lavi (2005)	• 740 Israeli youth (aged 11.5–15 years), including youth attending schools in settlements in the disputed territories (n = 307), youth living in a neighborhood of Jerusalem (n = 269), and youth living in the city of Jerusalem (n = 164)	• Data collection occurred during a period of ongoing conflict	• Exposure to terror events • PTSD Future orientation	• Exposure to terror events was positively associated with PTSD symptoms and openness to peace talks, but not with future orientation. • Youth living in settlements were more likely to report moderate to very severe PTSD symptoms than youth living in Jerusalem or a Jerusalem neighborhood • Approximately one-third of settlement-residing participants and half of participants residing in Jerusalem or a Jerusalem neighborhood supported the continuation of peace talks
Israel; Second Intifada	Cohen, Chazan, Lerner, and Maimon (2010)	• 54 Israeli youth, including youth who had and had not been directly exposed to terrorism (matched; M ages = 5.47 and 5.62 years, respectively)	• Data collection occurred during a period of ongoing conflict. The median elapsed time since exposure to terrorism for the exposed group was 15 months	• Exposure to traumatic events (caregiver report) • Play activity • PTSD (caregiver report) • Family background	• Among directly exposed participants, the types and severities of experienced traumatic events were reflected in posttraumatic play patterns. • Directly exposed participants exhibited higher rates of traumatic play activity, play interruptions, negative and trauma-related affects, and morbid play themes than non-exposed participants • Among directly exposed participants, posttraumatic play involving higher levels of "overwhelmed re-experiencing" coping strategies and lower levels of "reenactment with soothing" was positively associated with PTSD symptoms
Israel; Second Intifada	Slone and Shechner (2009)	• 3,667 Jewish Israeli youth (aged 10–18 years) sampled cross-sectionally at each time-point	• Baseline data collection occurred 0–2 years before the Intifada • T2 data collection occurred during the peak of the Intifada • T3 data collection occurred during the recession of the Intifada	• Political life events • Personal life events • Psychological symptoms	• Participants of all ages who reported high levels of exposure to political life events exhibited more severe psychological symptoms than participants with low levels of exposure For both genders, level of exposure to political life events was positively associated with the

(continued)

Table 4.1 (continued)

Region and conflict	Reference	Sample	Assessment Timing	Measures	Major Findings
					severity of psychological symptoms, but differed by time-point • Participants exhibited higher levels of psychological symptoms at T2 than either T1 or T3
Israel; Second Lebanon War	Schiff et al. (2010).	• 4,151 youth, including 1,800 Jewish Israelis and 2,351 Arab Israelis (grades 7–11)	• Data collection occurred 1 year after the war	• War exposure • PTSD • Perceived need for help • Preferred sources of help	• 7.4% of Arab participants and 3.5% of Jewish participants reported PTSD symptoms • Approximately one-third of participants reported needing help in the war's aftermath • Arab participants, females and participants with higher levels of PTSD symptoms were most likely to perceive that they needed help
Nepal; Nepalese Civil War	Kohrt et al. (2008)	• 282 youth (M age = 15.75 years), including former child soldiers and non-conscripted youth (matched; n = 141 and 141, respectively.)	• Data collection occurred 4–5 months after peace accords were signed	• Exposure to traumatic events • Depression • Anxiety • PTSD • General psychological difficulties • Daily functioning	• Former child soldiers exhibited worse mental health outcomes than non-conscripted participants, with the exception of anxiety symptoms • After controlling for traumatic exposure and other covariates, child soldier status was positively associated with depression and PTSD among girls, and with PTSD among boys • After controlling for traumatic exposure and other covariates, child soldier status was not significantly associated with general psychological difficulties, anxiety, or functional impairment
Palestine; Israeli–Palestinian Conflict	Abdeen, Qasrawi, Nabil, and Shaheen (2008)	• 2,100 Palestinian youth (M age = 15.9 years) from the West Bank (n = 1,235) and Gaza (n = 724)	• Data collection occurred during a period of ongoing conflict	• Exposure to traumatic events • Emotional reactions to trauma • PTSD • Functional impairment	• Exposure to violence was positively associated with PTSD symptoms and somatic complaints • Gazan youth self-reported significantly higher rates of PTSD symptoms than West Bank youth • Females reported significantly more somatic complaints than males

(continued)

Table 4.1 (continued)

Region and conflict	Reference	Sample	Assessment Timing	Measures	Major Findings
				• Hopelessness • Somatic complaints • Coping strategies	
Palestine; Israeli-Palestinian Conflict	Giacaman, Shannon, Saab, Arya, and Boyce (2007)	• 3,415 Palestinian youth (grades 10–11).	• Data collection occurred during a period of ongoing conflict • Participants were asked to report on experiences during army invasions from 1 year prior	• Individual exposure to trauma/violence • Collective exposure to violence • Depressive-like symptoms • Emotional problems • Somatic symptoms	• A strong positive relationship emerged between exposure to violence and psychological symptoms, with both individual and collective exposure exerting independent effects • Females reported significantly less exposure to violence, but significantly higher rates of depressive symptoms than males • Refugee camp dwellers reported significantly more depressive symptoms than participants living in cities, towns, or villages
Palestine; Second Intifada	Thabet, Abed, and Vostanis (2004).	• 403 youth living in refugee camps (M age = 12.0 years.)	• Data collection occurred during a period of ongoing conflict	• Exposure to traumatic events • PTSD • Depression	• Youth reported high exposure to traumatic events • High levels of traumatic exposure were positively associated with PTSD and depressive symptoms • Strong correlations emerged between participants' scores on measures of PTSD and depression, supporting a high degree of comorbidity
Europe					
Bosnia; Bosnian War	Allwood, Bell-Dolan, and Husain (2002)	• 791 Sarajevo youth (M age = 10.9 years).	• Data collection occurred during a period of ongoing conflict.	• War experiences • PTSD • Emotional and behavioral adjustment	• 41% of participants exhibited clinically significant PTSD symptoms • Exposure to both violent and nonviolent war traumas was significantly associated with significantly greater PTSD symptoms and adjustment problems

(continued)

Table 4.1 (continued)

Region and conflict	Reference	Sample	Assessment Timing	Measures	Major Findings
					• Cumulative trauma exposure exerted significant additive effects on adjustment problems
Bosnia and Herzegovina; Bosnian War	Goldstein et al (1997)	• 364 internally displaced youth and their parents (M youth age = years.)	• Data collection occurred during a period of ongoing conflict.	• Traumatic experiences • Psychological distress, including PTSD	• Participants reported high levels of traumatic exposure. • Almost 94% of participants exhibited clinical levels of PTSD symptoms • Participants also reported high levels of sadness, anxiety, and distress • Age, urban residence, and witnessing the injury, torture, or death of an immediate family member were associated with elevated symptomatology
Bosnia and Herzegovina; Croat-Bosniak War	Smith, Perrin, Yule, Hacam, and Stuvland (2002)	• 2,976 youth (M age = 12.11 years) living in a town heavily affected by the war	• Data collection occurred 2 years after the signing of a cease-fire agreement	• Exposure to traumatic war events • Impact of events • Depression • Anxiety Grief	• Participants reported high levels of PTSD and grief reactions; however, rates of anxiety and depression were not significantly elevated • Levels of exposure to war events were positively associated with levels of psychological distress • Certain types of war experiences (e.g., perceived direct life threat) were more strongly associated with psychological distress • Females reported significantly higher levels of psychological distress than males
Croatia; Croatian War of Independence	Brajša-Žganec (2005)	• 583 youth who had been displaced from their homes and were living in the Croatian capital (aged 12–15 years), including resident youth (n = 300) and youth from different towns (n = 283)	• Data collection occurred approximately three and a half years after participants were exposed to war events	• Exposure to traumatic war events • Depression • Extraversion • Interpersonal support	• Cumulative war experiences were positively associated with male depressive symptoms • Perceived interpersonal support was inversely associated with male depressive symptoms • Instrumental support and self-esteem levels were inversely associated with female depressive symptoms

(continued)

Table 4.1 (continued)

Region and conflict	Reference	Sample	Assessment Timing	Measures	Major Findings
Croatia; Croatian War of Independence	Vizek-Vidović, Kuterovac-Jagodić, and Arambašić (2000)	• 1,034 Croatian youth (M age = 11.56 years) living in towns severely affected by the war	• Data collection occurred during a period of ongoing conflict	• Exposure to traumatic war events • PTSD • Depression • Anxiety • Psychosomatic reactions • Psychosocial adaptation	• Cumulative traumatization was positively associated with rates of psychological symptoms • Younger children reported significantly more PTSD symptoms than older children • Among older children, females reported higher levels of PTSD, anxiety, and depression symptoms but also higher levels of psychosocial adaptation
Northern Ireland; the Troubles	McAloney, McCrystal, Percy, and McCartan (2009)	• 3,828 Belfast youth (aged 15–16 years)	• Data collection occurred after the Troubles, but during a period of ongoing tension.	• Experiences with community violence • Psychosis • Depression Substance misuse	• Over three quarters of participants reported exposure to community violence. Levels of community violence exposure were positively associated with depressive symptoms, psychotic symptoms, and substance misuse

Summary

Tier 1 research documents the links between exposure to political violence and youth adjustment, particularly internalizing and externalizing problems. These studies suggest that individual differences between youth (e.g., age and gender) matter, though their precise impact is unclear. Moreover, a limited number of studies in Tier 1 document how vulnerable youth may well exhibit resilience and grow into well-adjusted adulthood. This acknowledgment marks an important move away from previous conceptual frameworks that assumed universal maladjustment and traumatization among affected youth.

The studies that are presented in detail in Table 4.1 represent the diverse populations and regions that have been studied at the Tier 1 level, indicating the widespread effects of exposure to political violence on youth functioning. Among the strengths of studies in Table 4.1 are large samples, even when data collection occurred during ongoing conflict; explicit and diverse measures of youths' exposure to political violence; and a limited examination of some non-psychopathology-related outcomes. Limitations of Tier 1 studies include the cross-sectional characteristics of data collection and analyses; inability to eliminate third variable explanations or assess the direction of effects; and the absence of explicit measurement of mediators, process-oriented moderators, or social-ecological contexts.

An important point to emphasize in the Tier 1 literature is the heavy focus on psychopathology, including internalizing and externalizing problems. It is important for researchers to investigate a broad range of outcomes and areas of functioning relevant to youth and the contexts in which they live. Going beyond just the study of psychopathology, important developmental processes and outcomes to be considered might include peer relations, academic difficulties, romantic relationships, and identity development. As discussed below in the road map, we encourage researchers to think more broadly about domains of development that can be impacted by political conflict and armed violence.

This notion that we should broaden our scope of outcomes assessed is also motivated by debates about resilience. We echo Dawes, Tredoux, and Feinstein's (1989) and Betancourt and Khan's (2008) warnings that despite the importance of the construct of resilience, researchers should not be so seduced by its optimism. That is, we should not gloss over the serious developmental and psychological repercussions that political violence and armed conflict may inflict on youth. As we have discussed, published studies report the incidence and prevalence of clinical and subclinical mental health problems tends to be significant among youth who have been exposed to armed conflict compared to non-exposed peers (e.g., Attanayake et al., 2009). Yet, it is important to note, however, that effect sizes may be relatively small, and studies that do not find a significant link may not be published. Thus, a long-term goal must also be to promote healthier outcomes among this population, not simply avoiding adjustment problems, ideally by advancing research-guided prevention and intervention efforts for those at risk (Cummings, Davies, & Campbell, 2000).

Thus, while Tier 1 research firmly establishes the potential risks endured by youth exposed to multiple and diverse contexts of armed conflict as the base of the research pyramid, studies conducted at this level do not provide solid empirical support to inform the development of translational intervention efforts.

References

Abdeen, Z., Qasrawi, R., Nabil, S., & Shaheen, M. (2008). Psychological reactions to Israeli occupation: Findings from the national study of school-based screening in Palestine. *International Journal of Behavioral Development, 32*(4), 290–297. doi:10.1177/016502540809220.

Ahmad, A., von Knorring, A.-L., & Sundelin-Wahlstein, V. (2008). Traumatic experiences and post-traumatic stress symptoms in Kurdish children in their native country and in exile. *Child and Adolescent Mental Health, 13*(4), 193–197. doi:10.1111/j.1475-3588.2008.00501.x.

Alcock, A. T. (1941). War strain in children. *British Medical Journal, 1*(25), 124.

Al-Krenawi, A., & Graham, J. R. (2012). The impact of political violence on psychosocial functioning of individuals and families: The case of Palestinian adolescents. *Child and Adolescent Mental Health, 17*(1), 14–22. doi:10.1111/j.1475-3588.2011.00600.x.

Allwood, M. A., Bell-Dolan, D., & Husain, S. A. (2002). Children's trauma and adjustment reactions to violent and nonviolent war experiences. *Journal of the American Academy of Child and Adolescent Psychiatry, 41*(4), 450–457. doi:10.1097/00004583-200204000-00018.

Attanayake, V., McKay, R., Joffres, M., Singh, S., Burkle, F., & Mills, E. (2009). Prevalence of mental disorders among children exposed to war: A systematic review of 7,920 children. *Medicine, Conflict and Survival, 25*(1), 4–19. doi:10.1080/13623690802568913.

Barber, B. K. (2013). Political conflict and youth. *Psychologist, 26*(5), 336–339.

Betancourt, T. S., & Khan, K. T. (2008). The mental health of children affected by armed conflict: Protective processes and pathways to resilience. *International Review of Psychiatry, 20*(3), 317–328. doi:10.1080/09540260802090363.

Bodman, F. (1941). War conditions and the mental health of the child. *British Medical Journal, 2*(4213), 486–488.

Bodman, F. H., & Dunsdon, M. A. (1941). Juvenile delinquency in war-time: Report from the Bristol Child-Guidance Clinic. *The Lancet, 238*(6167), 572–574.

Brajša- Žganec, A. (2005). The long-term effects of war experiences on children's depression in the Republic of Croatia. *Child Abuse and Neglect, 29*(1), 31–43. doi:10.1016/j.chiabu.2004.07.007.

Burbury, W. M. (1941). Effects of evacuation and of air raids on city children. *British Medical Journal, 2*(4218), 660–662.

Burt, C. (1940). The incidence of neurotic symptoms among evacuated school children. *British Journal of Educational Psychology, 10*(1), 8–15. doi:10.1111/j.2044-8279.1940.tb02679.x.

Cohen, E., Chazan, S., Lerner, M., & Maimon, E. (2010). Posttraumatic play in young children exposed to terrorism: An empirical study. *Infant Mental Health Journal, 31*(2), 159–181. doi:10.1002/imhj.20250.

Cummings, E. M., Davies, P. T., & Campbell, S. B. (2000). *Developmental psychopathology and family process: Theory, research, and clinical implications*. New York: Guilford Press.

Dawes, A., Tredoux, C., & Feinstein, A. (1989). Political violence in South Africa: Some effects on children of the violent destruction of their community. *International Journal of Mental Health, 18*(2), 16–43.

Derluyn, I., Broekaert, E., Schuyten, G., & De Temmerman, E. (2004). Post-traumatic stress in former Ugandan child soldiers. *Lancet, 363*(9412), 861–863. doi:10.1016/S0140-6736(04)15734-6.

Despert, J. L. (1944). Effects of war on children's mental health. *Journal of Consulting Psychology, 8*(4), 206–218. doi:10.1037/h0054103.

Dimitry, L. (2011). A systematic review on the mental health of children and adolescents in areas of armed conflict in the Middle East. *Child: Care, Health, and Development, 38*(2), 153–161. doi:10.1111/j.1365-2214.2011.01246.x.

Dyregrov, A., Gupta, L., Gjestad, R., & Mukanoheli, E. (2000). Trauma exposure and psychological reactions to genocide among Rwandan children. *Journal of Traumatic Stress, 13*(1), 3–21. doi:10.1023/A:1007759112499.

Fazel, M., Reed, R. V., Panter-Brick, C., & Stein, A. (2012). Mental health of displaced and refugee children resettled in high-income countries: Risk and protective factors. *The Lancet, 379*(9812), 266–282. doi:10.1016/S0140-6736(11)60051-2.

Freud, A., & Burlingham, D. T. (1943). *War and children*. New York, NY: International University Press.

Giacaman, R., Shannon, H. S., Saab, H., Arya, N., & Boyce, W. (2007). Individual and collective exposure to political violence: Palestinian adolescents coping with conflict. *European Journal of Public Health, 17*(4), 361–368. doi:10.1093/curpub/ckl260.

Goldstein, R. D., Wampler, N. S., & Wise, P. H. (1997). War experiences and distress symptoms of Bosnian children. *Pediatrics, 100*(5), 873–878. doi:10.1542/peds.100.5.873.

John, E. M. (1941). A study of the effects of evacuation and air raids on children of pre-school age. *British Journal of Educational Psychology, 11*, 173–182.

Kasler, J., Dahan, J., & Elias, M. J. (2008). The relationship between sense of hope, family support and post-traumatic stress disorder among children: The case of young victims of rocket attacks in Israel. *Vulnerable Children and Youth Studies, 3*(3), 182–191. doi:10.1080/17450120802282876.

Klasen, F., Oettingen, G., Daniels, J., & Adams, H. (2010). Multiple trauma and mental health in former Ugandan child soldiers. *Journal of Traumatic Stress, 23*(5), 573–581. doi:10.1002/jts.20557.

Kohrt, B. A., Jordans, M. J. D., Tol, W. A., Speckman, R. A., Maharjan, S. M., Worthman, C. M., … & Komproe, I. H. (2008). Comparison of mental health between former child soldiers and children never conscripted by armed groups in Nepal. *JAMA, 300*(6), 691–702. doi:10.1001/jama.300.6.691.

Lev-Wiesel, R., Al-Krenawi, A., & Schwail, M. A. (2007). Psychological symptomatology among Palestinian male and female adolescents living under political violence 2004–2005. *Community Mental Health Journal, 43*(1), 49–56. doi:10.1007/s10597-006-9060-9.

McAloney, K., McCrystal, P., Percy, A., & McCartan, C. (2009). Damaged youth: Prevalence of community violence exposure and implications for adolescent wellbeing in post-conflict Northern Ireland. *Journal of Community Psychology, 37*(5), 635–648. doi:10.1002/jcop.20322.

Miller, T., El-Masri, M., Allodi, F., & Qouta, S. (1999). Emotional and behavioural problems and trauma exposure of school-age Palestinian children in Gaza: Some preliminary findings. *Medicine, Conflict, and Survival, 15*(4), 368–378, 391–393. doi:10.1080/13623699908409478.

Mollica, R. F., Poole, C., Son, L., Murray, C. C., & Tor, S. (1997). Effects of war trauma on Cambodian refugee adolescents' functional health and mental health status. *Journal of the American Academy of Child and Adolescent Psychiatry, 36*(8), 1098–1106. doi:10.1097/00004583-199708000-00017.

Morgos, D., Worden, J. R., & Gupta, L. (2007). Psychosocial effects of war experiences among displaced children in Southern Darfur. *Omega—Journal of Death and Dying, 56*(3), 229–253. doi:10.2190/OM.56.3b.

Okello, J., De Schryver, M., Musisi, S., Broekaert, E., & Derluyn, I. (2014). Differential roles of childhood adversities and stressful war experiences in the development of mental health symptoms in post-war adolescents in northern Uganda. *BMC Psychiatry, 14*, 260. doi:10.1186/s12888-014-0260-5.

Okello, J., Onen, T. S., & Musisi, S. (2007). Psychiatric disorders among war-abducted and non-abducted adolescents in Gulu district, Uganda: A comparative study. *African Journal of Psychiatry, 10*(4), 225–231. doi:10.4314/ajpsy.v10i4.30260.

Paardekooper, B., de Jong, J. T. V. M., & Hermanns, J. M. A. (1999). The psychological impact of war and the refugee situation on South Sudanese children in refugee camps in Northern Uganda: An exploratory study. *Journal of Child Psychology and Psychiatry, 40*(4), 529–536.

Punamäki, R.-L. (1996). Can ideological commitment protect children's psychosocial wellbeing in situations of political violence? *Child Development, 67*(1), 55–69. doi:10.1111/j.1467-8624.1996.tb01719.x.

Ronen, T., Rahav, G., & Appel, N. (2003). Adolescent stress responses to a single acute stress and to continuous external stress: Terrorist attacks. *Journal of Loss and Trauma, 8*(4), 261–282. doi:10.1080/15325020390233075.

Rosenblatt, R. (1983). *Children of war.* New York: Anchor Press/Doubleday.

Sack, W. H., Clarke, G. N., & Seeley, J. (1996). Multiple forms of stress in Cambodian adolescent refugees. *Child Development, 67*(1), 107–116. doi:10.1111/j.1467-8624.1996.tb01722.x.

Sagi-Schwartz, A. (2008). The well being of children living in chronic war zones: The Palestinian-Israeli case. *International Journal of Behavioral Development, 32*(4), 322–336. doi:10.1177/0165025408090974.

Schiff, M., Benbenishty, R., McKay, M., DeVoe, E., Liu, X., & Hasin, D. (2006). Exposure to terrorism and Israeli youths' psychological distress and alcohol use: An exploratory study. *The American Journal on Addictions, 15*(3), 220–226. doi:10.1080/10550490600626200.

Schiff, M., Pat-Horenczyk, R., Benbenishty, R., Brom, D., Baum, N., & Astor, R. A. (2010). Do adolescents know when they need help in the aftermath of war? *Journal of Traumatic Stress, 23*(5), 657–660. doi:10.1002/jts.20558.

Schwarzwald, J., Weisenberg, M., Waysman, M., Solomon, Z., & Klingman, A. (1993). Stress reaction of school-age children to the bombardment by SCUD missiles. *Journal of Abnormal Psychology, 102*(3), 404–410. doi:10.1037/0021-843X.102.3.404.

Shaw, J. A. (2003). Children exposed to war/terrorism. *Clinical Child and Family Psychology Review, 6*(4), 237–246. doi:10.1023/B:CCFP.0000006291.10180.bd.

Slone, M., Kaminer, D., & Durrheim, K. (2000). The contribution of political life events to psychological distress among South African adolescents. *Political Psychology, 21*(3), 465–487. doi:10.1111/0162-895X.00199.

Slone, M., & Shechner, T. (2009). Psychiatric consequences for Israeli adolescents of protracted political violence: 1998–2004. *Journal of Child Psychology and Psychiatry, 50*(3), 280–289. doi:10.1111/j.1469-7610.2008.01940.x.

Smith, P., Perrin, S., Yule, W., Hacam, B., & Stuvland, R. (2002). War exposure among children from Bosnia-Hercegovina: Psychological adjustment in a community sample. *Journal of Traumatic Stress, 15*(2), 147–156. doi:10.1023/A:1014812209051.

Solomon, Z., & Lavi, T. (2005). Israeli youth in the second intifada: PTSD and future orientation. *Journal of the American Academy of Child and Adolescent Psychiatry, 44*(11), 1167–1175. doi:10.1097/01.chi.0000161650.97643.e1.

Thabet, A. A. M., Abed, Y., & Vostanis, P. (2004). Comorbidity of PTSD and depression among refugee children during war conflict. *Journal of Child Psychology and Psychiatry, 45*(3), 533–542. doi:10.1111/j.1469-7610.2004.00243.x.

Tolley, H. (1973). *Political socialization to international conflict.* New York: Teachers' College Press.

Vizek-Vidović, V., Kuterovac-Jagodić, G., & Arumbašić, L. (2000). Posttraumatic symptomatology in children exposed to war. *Scandinavian Journal of Psychology, 41*(4), 297–306. doi:10.1111/1467-9450.00202.

Young, F. M. (1947). Psychological effects of war on young children. *American Journal of Orthopsychiatry, 17*(3), 500–510. doi:10.1111/j.1939-0025.1947.tb05024.x.

Ziv, A., & Israel, R. (1973). Effects of bombardment on the manifest anxiety level of children living in kibbutzim. *Journal of Counseling and Clinical Psychology, 40,* 287–291.

Ziv, A., Kruglanski, A. W., & Shulman, S. (1974). Children's psychological reactions to wartime stress. *Journal of Personality and Social Psychology, 30,* 24–30.

Chapter 5
Tier 2: Cross-Sectional Studies of Mediators, Process-Oriented Moderators, and Social-Ecological Contexts

Keywords Cross-sectional mediation and moderators · Risk and protective processes · Cognitive appraisal · Coping strategies · Ideological meaning · Parent–child relationship

Tier 2 research as we define it expands beyond Tier 1 by exploring factors that moderate, and potentially mediate, the effects of armed conflict on youth adjustment in multiple contexts (see Fig. 3.1). Unlike Tier 1 studies, which focus on the contributions of demographic variables (e.g., age and gender), Tier 2 includes exploration of psychological and social variables (e.g., coping strategies and family dynamics).

In the course of our review, we identified approximately 95 studies that fit the criteria for Tier 2. We will now discuss noteworthy findings and patterns from this body of work. We also selected a diverse subset of Tier 2 studies ($N = 20$) according to the previously discussed criteria and have presented them in detail in Table 5.1. As with Table 4.1, Table 5.1 should not be interpreted as a definitive list of Tier 2 studies. Rather, it should be viewed in light of the goal of representing the depth and breadth of work conducted at the Tier 2 level.

Investigating Multiple Levels of the Social Ecology

By our definition, Tier 2 research provides a stronger foundation for subsequent translational research by more closely examining the effects of armed conflict on youth functioning in the *contexts* of the family, school, community, and culture (Cummings, Goeke-Morey, Merrilees, Taylor, & Shirlow, 2014). Youth who have been exposed to political violence are at increased odds of maladjustment, and this risk is often further exacerbated by stressors in other domains that may or may not be directly related to the conflict (e.g., poverty following displacement and marital conflict). Likewise, youths' probabilities of maintaining competent functioning in the face of conflict may be enhanced by adaptive systems and protective processes that are embedded in their environments.

© Springer International Publishing AG 2017
E.M. Cummings et al., *Political Violence, Armed Conflict, and Youth Adjustment*,
DOI 10.1007/978-3-319-51583-0_5

Table 5.1 *Tier 2*

Region and conflict	Reference	Sample	Assessment timing	Measures	Major findings
AFRICA					
Sierra Leone; Sierra Leonean Civil War	Newnham, Pearson, Stein, and Betancourt (2015)	• 363 youth who reported at least one war exposure, including former child soldiers who received disarmament, demobilization, and reintegration services postwar; former child soldiers who did not receive services; and a community sample of war-affected youth	• Data collection occurred six years after the war	• Exposure to traumatic war events • Daily stressors • PTSD • Depression	• Level of war exposure was positively associated with PTSD symptoms, and a significant proportion of this relationship was explained by indirect pathways through daily stressors • The relationship between level of war exposure and depression symptoms was completely explained by indirect pathways through daily stressors
ASIA					
Afghanistan; ongoing conflict	Panter-Brick, Eggerman, Gonzalez, and Safdar (2009)	• 1,011 youth (*M* age = 13.5 years), caregivers and teachers	• Data collection occurred during a period of ongoing conflict	• Youth exposure to traumatic events • Youth impact of traumatic events • Youth depression • Youth behavioral, emotional, and social problems • Caregiver exposure to traumatic events • Caregiver mental health	• Female gender, exposure to five or more traumatic events, caregiver mental health, and residence area were positively associated with probable psychiatric ratings and depressive symptoms • Age, exposure to five or more traumatic events, and caregiver mental health were significantly associated with PTSD symptoms

(continued)

Table 5.1 (continued)

Region and conflict	Reference	Sample	Assessment timing	Measures	Major findings
Israel; Israeli–Palestinian Conflict	Feldman, Vengrover, Eidelman-Rothman, and Zagoory-Sharon (2013)	• 232 mother–child dyads (M youth age = 33.08 months), including dyads living in an area heavily affected by the war (n = 148) and dyads living in an area not affected by acts of political violence during the study period (n = 84)	• Data collection occurred during a period of ongoing conflict in the area where the 148-dyad subsample lived	• Youth and family exposure to trauma • Youth PTSD • Youth fear regulation • Youth cortisol and salivary alpha amylase levels • Mother–child reciprocity • Maternal PTSD • Maternal cortisol and salivary alpha amylase levels	• Maternal cortisol, maternal PTSD, low mother–child reciprocity, and negative emotionality predicted child cortisol levels • Youth with PTSD exhibited significantly lower levels of cortisol and salivary alpha amylase • Youth who had been exposed to traumatic war events, but who did not report PTSD symptoms exhibited significantly higher levels of cortisol and salivary alpha amylase • Youth who had been exposed to traumatic war events exhibited higher levels of negative emotionality • Youth who had been exposed to traumatic war events, but who did not report PTSD symptoms tended to employ comfort-seeking strategies, whereas exposed youth with PTSD tended to employ withdrawal strategies

(continued)

Table 5.1 (continued)

Region and conflict	Reference	Sample	Assessment timing	Measures	Major findings
					• Youth who had not been exposed to traumatic war events displayed low salivary alpha amylase, increases in cortisol following challenge, and reductions in cortisol upon recovery from challenge
Israel; Israeli-Palestinian Conflict	Lavi and Slone (2011)	• 212 mother–child dyads from Jewish Israeli families ($n = 104$) and Arab Israeli families ($n = 108$) (M youth age = 10.73 years)	• Data collection occurred during a period of ongoing conflict	• Exposure to political life events (youth report) • Exposure to stressful life events (youth report) • Self-esteem (youth report) • Self-control (youth report) • Social difficulties (youth and mother reports) • Psychological problems (youth and mother reports)	• High levels of political life events were positively associated with social, psychological, and behavioral problems among Arab, but not Jewish, youth • Self-control moderated the link between political life events and Jewish youths' problems • Self-esteem moderated the link between political life events and Arab youths' problems

(continued)

Table 5.1 (continued)

Region and conflict	Reference	Sample	Assessment timing	Measures	Major findings
				• Behavioral problems (youth and mother reports)	
Israel; Israeli–Palestinian Conflict	Slone, Lobel, and Gilat (1999)	• 397 Israeli youth (aged 12–13 years), including youth from West Bank settlements (n = 159), Golan Heights (n = 71), and the greater Tel Aviv area (n = 167)	• Data collection occurred during a period of strained peace negotiations	• Exposure to political life events • Impact of political life events • Psychological symptoms • Perception of threat • Ideological commitment	• Impact of political life events and perception of threat were positively associated with levels of psychological distress • Ideological commitment did not mediate the relationship between psychopolitical variables and psychological distress
Israel; Second Intifada	Laufer and Solomon (2011)	• 1,973 non-secular youth (aged 13–15 years) living in the areas affected by low and high levels of terror	• Data collection occurred during a period of ongoing conflict	• Objective and subjective exposure to war and terror • PTSD • Religious orientation	• Objective and subjective terror exposure, personal extrinsic orientations, and social extrinsic orientations were positively associated with PTSD symptoms • Intrinsic religiosity was negatively associated with PTSD symptoms
Israel and Palestine; Second Intifada	Al-Krenawi, Graham, and Kanat-Maymon (2009)	• 892 youth (aged 14–18 years), including Israeli Jews (n = 442) and Palestinians (n = 450)	• Data collection occurred during a period of ongoing conflict	• Exposure to political violence • Psychological symptoms	• Palestinian participants reported higher levels of exposure to political violence, psychological symptoms, PTSD symptoms,

(continued)

Table 5.1 (continued)

Region and conflict	Reference	Sample	Assessment timing	Measures	Major findings
				• PTSD • Aggression • Social functioning • Family functioning	aggression, social functioning problems, and family functioning problems than Israeli participants • Females reported higher levels of psychological and PTSD symptoms • Males reported higher levels of aggression and family functioning problems • Participants with more social functioning problems also reported more psychological and PTSD symptoms • Lower socioeconomic status was associated with higher levels of psychological and PTSD symptoms, and social and family functioning problems
Israel; ongoing terror attacks.	Laor et al. (2006)	• 1,105 youth (M age = 14.6 years) from schools exposed to continuous terrorism	• Data collection occurred during a period of ongoing conflict	• War-related traumatic experiences • Non-war-related traumatic experiences • PTSD	• Trauma exposure levels were positively associated with psychological symptoms • Trauma exposure levels were inversely related to levels of personal resilience

(continued)

Table 5.1 (continued)

Region and conflict	Reference	Sample	Assessment timing	Measures	Major findings
				• Traumatic dissociation and grief • Personal resilience • Willingness to make sacrifices for one's country • Family willingness to discuss terror attacks	• Perceived personal resilience was inversely related to psychological symptoms
Israel; ongoing terror attacks	Laufer, Raz-Hamama, Levine, and Solomon (2009)	• 1,482 youth (age 16 years), including religious Jews (n = 181), traditional Jews (n = 515), and secular Jews (n = 772)	• Data collection occurred following terror attacks	• Exposure to terror attacks • Negative life events • PTSD • Post-traumatic growth • Forgiveness	• Religious participants reported higher levels of post-traumatic growth than secular participants • Among secular and traditional participants, PTSD, and unwillingness to forgive were positively associated with post-traumatic growth • Fear of terror was positively associated with post-traumatic growth in all groups
Israel and Palestine; Israeli–Palestinian Conflict	Harel-Fisch et al. (2010)	• 24,935 youth (aged 11, 13, and 15 years), including West Bank Palestinians (n = 7,430), Gaza residents (n = 7,217), Israeli	• Data collection occurred during a period of ongoing conflict	• Exposure to armed conflict • Subjective threat from armed conflict	• Subjective threat from armed conflict events was associated with negative mental health outcomes, diminished well-being, and elevated risk

(continued)

Table 5.1 (continued)

Region and conflict	Reference	Sample	Assessment timing	Measures	Major findings
		Jews ($n = 5,255$), and Arab Israelis ($n = 6,033$)		• PTSD • Life satisfaction • Positive health perceptions • Smoking • Involvement in youth violence • Parental support	behaviors across all four populations. Effects were strongest among Israeli Jews and weakest among Arab Israelis • Parental support exerted a significant main effect on all outcome variables and buffered the effects of subjective threat from armed conflict events on PTSD symptoms, life satisfaction, positive life perceptions, and tobacco use
Kuwait; Gulf War	Llabre and Hadi (1997)	• 151 Kuwaiti youth (M age = 10.5 years), including youth who were exposed to high levels of war trauma ($n = 112$) and youth who were exposed to relatively low levels of war trauma ($n = 39$)	• Data collection occurred 2 years after the war	• PTSD • Depression • Social support • Health complaints	• High levels of trauma were associated with higher levels of PTSD symptoms, depressive symptoms, and health complaints • The relationship between trauma and distress was jointly moderated by gender and social support • Females reported higher levels of social support than males, and social support buffered the effects of trauma among females only

(continued)

Table 5.1 (continued)

Region and conflict	Reference	Sample	Assessment timing	Measures	Major findings
Lebanon and Gaza Strip; ongoing conflict	Khamis (2012)	• 600 youth from highly war-exposed areas, including youth from South Lebanon (M age = 14.15 years; n = 300) and the Gaza Strip (M age = 12.83 years; n = 300)	• Data collection occurred during a period of ongoing conflict	• Trauma exposure • PTSD • Depression and anxiety • Economic pressure • Religiosity • Ideological commitment	• High levels of economic pressure were associated with higher rates of PTSD symptoms and psychological distress, especially among Gaza participants • Among Gaza participants, religiosity was positively associated with depression and anxiety symptoms • Among Lebanese participants, religiosity exerted a protective effect against depression and anxiety symptoms • Among Gaza participants, ideology was negatively associated with depression and anxiety symptoms • Among Lebanese participants, ideology was not significantly related to depression or anxiety symptoms
Nepal; Nepalese Civil War	Kohrt et al. (2010)	• 142 former child soldiers (M age = 15.75 years)	• The number of months since return to the community ranged from 1 to 62 at the time of data collection	• Traumatic life events • PTSD • Depression • Functional impairment	• High levels of trauma exposure were associated with poor psychosocial outcomes • High levels of education were associated with better psychosocial outcomes

(continued)

Table 5.1 (continued)

Region and conflict	Reference	Sample	Assessment timing	Measures	Major findings
				• Reintegration supports and difficulties • Family structure • Family dynamics • Family traumas • Community conflict mortality • Community literacy levels • Community caste system prevalence	• Conflict-related death of a relative, physical abuse in the household, and conflict-related loss of wealth predicted poor family functioning • Youth living in high-caste communities reported the lowest levels of reintegration support
Palestine; First Intifada	Barber (2001)	• 6,000 refugee and non-refugee Palestinian youth (aged 14 years), including West Bank refugees, Gaza Strip refugees, and Gaza Strip non-refugees	• Data collection occurred 1–2 years after the end of the Intifada	• Intifada experiences • Depression • Antisocial behavior • Educational experiences • Religious beliefs and behaviors • Peer relations • Perceived quality of the parent–child relationship • Perceived parental	• Intifada experience was positively associated with religiosity • Among females, Intifada experience was positively associated with depression and antisocial behavior • Intifada experience was not significantly related to social integration in school, family, or peer relations • Neighborhood disorganization was the most consistent and powerful moderator of the relationship between Intifada

Table 5.1 (continued)

Region and conflict	Reference	Sample	Assessment timing	Measures	Major findings
				psychological control • Perceived parental behavioral control • Perceived parental support • Perceived social disorganization in the community	experience and youth problem behaviors
Palestine; Second Intifada	Peltonen, Qouta, El Sarraj, and Punamäki (2010)	• 227 youth α(M age = 11.37 years)	• Data collection occurred in the year after the end of the Intifada	• Military trauma • Depression • Psychological distress • Peer relations • Sibling relations	• Military trauma exposure was associated with intensive sibling rivalry and low friendship quality, especially among girls and younger youth • Sibling rivalry and low friendship quality mediated the relationship between military trauma exposure and psychological symptoms • Warm sibling relations moderated the negative effects of military trauma on psychological well-being
Palestine; Second		• Two samples	• Data collection occurred during a	• Exposure to military violence	• In Study 1, witnessing severe military violence was positively

(continued)

Table 5.1 (continued)

Region and conflict	Reference	Sample	Assessment timing	Measures	Major findings
Intifada (Study 2)	Qouta, Punamäki, Miller, and El Sarraj (2008)	• 640 youth (*M* age = 10.51 years), parents, and teachers in Study 1 • 225 youth (*M* age = 11.37 years) in Study 2	• period of relatively low violence in Study 1 • Data collection occurred during a period of high violence in Study 2 • Approximately 8 years elapsed between studies	(parent report in Study 1; youth report in Study 2) • Aggressiveness (youth, parent, and teacher report in Study 1; youth report in Study 2) • Parenting practices (youth and parent reports in Study 1; not assessed in Study 2)	associated with aggressive and antisocial behaviors • In Study 1, the relations between exposure to military violence and aggressive behavior were moderated by supportive parenting practices • In Study 2, witnessing severe military violence was positively associated with proactive and reactive aggression and aggression enjoyment
EUROPE					
Bosnia; Bosnian War	Duraković-Belko, Kulenović, and Đapić (2003)	• 393 youth (*M* age = 17.0 years)	• Data collection occurred after the war ended	• Traumatic war experiences • PTSD • Depression • Extraversion • Life orientations • Perceived incompetence • Perceived social support • Cognitive appraisals	• Traumatic war experiences, personality characteristics, cognitive appraisals, and coping mechanisms were significantly associated with PTSD symptoms • Individual and socio-environmental factors (e.g., female gender and low optimism) were strongly associated with depressive symptoms

(continued)

Table 5.1 (continued)

Region and conflict	Reference	Sample	Assessment timing	Measures	Major findings
				• Coping mechanisms	• War trauma dimensions were also associated with depressive symptoms
Bosnia; Bosnian War	Jones and Kafetsios (2005)	• 337 youth from two cities on the opposite sides of the war (aged 13–15 years)	• Data collection occurred 2–3 years after the conflict ended	• Exposure to traumatic war events • Subjective psychological well-being • Academic grades	• Relations between traumatic war exposure, displacement, and psychological well-being varied based on the residential location • Specific meanings attributed to different war events moderated the relations between traumatic war exposure and youth outcomes • Worrying about school performance, missing friends, and breakdown of the family also exerted significant effects on psychological well-being
Chechnya; Second Chechen War	Betancourt et al. (2012)	• 183 internally displaced youth (M age = 13.6 years)	• Data collection occurred during a period of ongoing conflict	• War-related stressors • Emotional and behavioral problems Connectedness	• Female participants reported more emotional and behavioral problems than males • Positive family relations, positive peer relations, and community connectedness were negatively associated with internalizing problems • Family connectedness exerted a significant protective effect

(continued)

Table 5.1 (continued)

Region and conflict	Reference	Sample	Assessment timing	Measures	Major findings
					against internalizing problems, above and beyond the contributions of age, gender, housing status, and other forms of support; this effect was strongest among males
Croatia; War in Croatia	Kereteš (2006)	• 694 youth (*M* age = 13.58 years) and their teachers, including residents of a town that was severely affected by the war (*n* = 349) and residents of a town that was less severely affected (*n* = 345)	• Data collection occurred several years after the war ended	• War experiences (youth report) • Aggressive behavior (youth, peer, and teacher reports) • Prosocial behavior (youth, peer, and teacher reports) • Perceived parental behavior (youth report)	• Cumulative traumatic war experiences were associated with higher levels of self- and teacher-reported aggression and lower levels of teacher-rated prosocial behavior • Perceived positive parenting did not exert a protective effect on the relationship between cumulative trauma experiences and aggression • Among youth who positively perceived parenting behaviors, cumulative traumatic experiences were not associated with teacher-rated prosocial behaviors • Among youth who negatively perceived parenting behaviors, cumulative traumatic experiences were associated with lower teacher-rated prosocial behavior

Bronfenbrenner's (1979, 1986) ecological systems theory offers a valuable conceptual framework for studying broader environmental contexts and the psychological processes with which youth engage. This conceptual model has been frequently referenced in Tier 2 studies and involves five nested systems of varying degrees of influence and proximity to the developing individual. The first system, the *microsystem*, includes the individual and organizations which are most physically and psychologically proximal to him or her (e.g., family, school, and neighborhood.) The second system, the *mesosystem*, is comprised of the connections between the various microsystems within an individual's social ecology. The third system, the *exosystem*, includes environments which affect, or are affected by, the life experiences of the individual, but within which he or she does not actively participate (e.g., parents' workplaces). The fourth system, the *macrosystem*, subsumes the broader culture in which an individual lives (e.g., political or religious ideologies and systems). The final system, the *chronosystem*, contains major events and transitions in the life of an individual and his or her broader social-ecological contexts (e.g., death of a parent and the beginning of a war).

In contexts of political violence and armed conflict, risk and protective processes interplay at multiple social-ecological levels to shape youth development (Elbedour, ten Bensel, & Bastien, 1993; Tol, Song, & Jordans, 2013). Notably, youths' functioning levels may vary somewhat in different contexts, depending on how severely each context has been affected by conflict and on the unique supports and challenges present within them (Ungar, 2015). For these reasons, researchers aiming to capture a more comprehensive picture of the experiences of youth affected by political violence should ideally conduct their investigations across multiple levels of the social ecology (e.g., Dubow et al., 2010; Furr, Comer, Edmunds, & Kendall, 2010). Designing and carrying out such work are often very challenging and may require interdisciplinary collaboration.

We will now discuss the key findings and patterns from Tier 2, organized by levels of the social ecology.

Individual characteristics. Tier 2 studies have examined a wide range of individual-level variables as potential moderators or mediators of the effects of political violence on youth adjustment (e.g., see Table 5.1). Importantly, unlike Tier 1 studies, which primarily focus on individual demographic characteristics (e.g., age and gender), studies at the Tier 2 level have often examined individual psychological factors relevant to youth adjustment. Here, we will briefly review the findings on two major categories of individual characteristics: cognitive appraisals and coping styles, and ideological commitment.

Many Tier 2 studies have explored how youth cognitively appraise and cope in the settings of political violence and whether these processes moderate or mediate the relationship between exposure to violence and adjustment. For example, in a cross-sectional study of war-affected youth in Bosnia, Duraković-Belko, Kulenović, and Đapić (2003) reported that youths' cognitive appraisals (e.g., perceived meaningfulness of and control over war experiences) and coping mechanisms were significantly associated with PTSD symptoms. Meanwhile, in another study examining the cognitive appraisals in Israel, Sagy (2006) compared two cross-sectional samples of youth: one assessed during a chronic-without-acute-stress period (mid-Intifada) and one assessed during a chronic-with-acute-stress period (mid-Intifada, immediately after the assassination of a prime minister). Results indicated that youths' cognitive appraisals of the political situation significantly buffered the negative effects of stress on state anxiety among the chronic-without-acute-stress, but not chronic-with-acute-stress, sample.

In regard to coping strategies, Punamäki, Muhammed, and Abdulrahman (2004) evaluated the effectiveness of different coping strategies in buffering the mental health of Kurdish youth. They reported that the effectiveness of different coping dimensions (reconstructing, active affiliation, passivity, and denial) differed by symptom type (PTSD, sleeping problems, aggressive behavior). For example, active affiliation buffered the negative effects of traumatic events on post-traumatic symptoms and sleeping difficulties. Other studies have suggested that coping strategies and effectiveness may differ by youth gender, age, and conflict intensity. For example, in a study comparing cross-sectional samples of Palestinian youth tested before and during the Intifada, Punamäki and Puhakka (1997) reported that older youth used wider coping repertoires, including more emotional and cognitive coping, than younger ones. In this study, boys were more likely to use problem restructuring and behavioral coping strategies than girls, who used more emotional coping strategies. There was also evidence that youths' coping repertoires narrowed during the periods of intensive conflict and that certain coping strategies buffered against psychosocial problems during, but not before, the Intifada (e.g., problem restructuring, active fighting, and behavioral coping). Taken together, this body of findings points to the importance of carefully assessing how different groups of youth (e.g., age, gender, and nationality) cognitively appraise and emotionally cope with different experiences of political violence and of assessing how effective different appraisal and coping styles are in promoting youth adjustment.

Youth ideological commitments (religious and political) have also been commonly studied at the Tier 2 level, with mixed findings. Some studies have reported that high levels of religious or political commitment exert protective effects on youth adjustment in contexts of political violence. For example, in a study examining psychopathology among war-affected Israeli youth, Laufer and Solomon (2011) reported that intrinsic religiosity was negatively associated with PTSD symptoms. Meanwhile, in a cross-sectional study comparing the psychological adjustment of religious, traditional, and secular Jewish youth in Israel, religious participants exhibited higher levels of post-traumatic growth (e.g., increased personal strength and appreciation for life) than secular ones (Laufer, Raz-Hamama, Levine, & Solomon, 2009).

Other studies have reported negative or mixed findings on the effects of ideological commitment on youth adjustment in contexts of political violence. For example, in a cross-sectional study in Israel, Slone, Lobel, and Gilat (1999) reported that political–religious ideological commitments did not mediate the relationship between exposure to political life events and youth psychological distress. Meanwhile, Khamis (2012) reported mixed findings from a cross-sectional study comparing war-affected youth from South Lebanon and the Gaza Strip. In this study, religiosity emerged as a risk factor for depression and anxiety among Gazan participants, but as a protective factor for Lebanese participants. Meanwhile, ideological commitment emerged as a protective factor for depression and anxiety among Gazan participants, but was not significantly related to Lebanese participants' symptoms. In another study with mixed findings, Schiff (2006) compared the psychological outcomes of religious and non-religious Jewish youth in Jerusalem. In this study, religious youth reported greater exposure to terrorism, but lower levels of PTSD and alcohol consumption than non-religious participants. Among religious participants only, problem-solving coping skills predicted higher levels of depressive symptoms. Meanwhile, emotion-focused coping styles predicted higher levels of alcohol consumption among non-religious participants with high levels of terrorism exposure, as well as among religious participants with low levels of exposure. These results underscore the importance of examining how multiple individual characteristics may interact to influence youth adjustment.

Tier 2 research, including the studies that have been reviewed above and those presented in Table 5.1, has valuably identified a number of individual factors that may moderate the relationship between exposure to political violence and youth adjustment. Cognitive appraisal and coping styles, religiosity, and political ideology are among the most commonly studied factors and, given additional research, may be effective targets for intervention. However, these findings must be interpreted with caution given the cross-sectional design of Tier 2 studies, which prevents the identification of temporal relations between variables or causal processes. Additional longitudinal research is needed to replicate and expand upon Tier 2 findings on individual factors that contribute to youth adjustment in contexts of political violence.

Microsystem factors. Family variables are among the most commonly studied microsystem elements in the Tier 2 literature. Regarding the nuclear family, quality of perceived parenting, parental mental health, perceived family support, and family conflict have been studied. For example, whereas warm, supportive, and non-punitive parenting behaviors have been linked to more positive youth adjustment in the face of violent conflict, inconsistent parenting, and high levels of parental psychological control have been linked to higher rates of psychological symptoms (e.g., Barber, 1999; Keresteŝ, 2006; Punamäki, Quota, & El-Sarraj, 2001; Thabet, Ibraheem, Shivram, Winter, & Vostanis, 2009). Significant positive relationships have also emerged between the mental health statuses of parents and their children (e.g., Almqvist & Broberg, 1999; Joshi & O'Donnell, 2003; Merrilees et al., 2011; Smith, Perrin, Yule, & Rabe-Hesketh, 2001). Beyond the parent–child relationship, family cohesion and functioning have been identified as regulators of youth adjustment, with perceived family support conferring protection and frequent family conflict conferring greater risk of psychological maladjustment (e.g., Al-Krenawi, Slonim-Nevo, Maymon, & Al-Krenawi, 2001; Laor, Wolmer, & Cohen, 2001). Taken together, these findings suggest that whereas positive parent–child and family relationships may serve as secure, protective bases for youth exposed to political violence, negative or unstable family relationships may further exacerbate their risk of maladjustment.

In regard to social relationships beyond the nuclear family, peer relations and perceived support are among the most commonly studied factors in Tier 2. For example, perceived acceptance and social support from friends and community members have frequently been identified as protective factors for youth affected by violent conflict (e.g., Betancourt, Brennan, Rubin-Smith, Fitzmaurice, & Gilman, 2010; Dimitry, 2011; O'Donnell, Schwab-Stone, & Muveed, 2002; Peltonen, Quota, El-Sarraj, & Punamäki, 2010; Shahar, Cohen, Grogan, Barile, & Henrich, 2009).

Summary

The Tier 2 literature begins painting a more comprehensive picture of the adjust-ment of youth exposed to political violence. This is accomplished by providing cross-sectional evidence for moderating, and potentially mediating, processes at multiple social-ecological levels (e.g., family, school, and community). Tier 2 studies thus provide further clarity regarding the factors and contexts that influence the youths' probabilities of arriving at negative or resilient outcomes.

Despite these strengths, Tier 2 research is methodologically and statistically limited in its ability to advance knowledge about youths' long-term adjustment in violent contexts. Studies at this level simultaneously measure exposure to violence and adjustment outcome using cross-sectional designs, providing only a snapshot of these variables at one particular time-point and developmental stage. Thus, Tier 2 studies can shed light on the associations among variables, but not on their temporal relations or the causal risk and protective processes that link them together.

Finally, Table 5.1 documents in rich detail the diversity of approaches and geographic regions that have been studied at the Tier 2 level, including research exploring psychological and social moderators, potential mediators, multiple con-texts, and other possible causal processes for the impact of political violence on children. Strengths of this body of studies include the often large sample sizes, even when data collection occurred during periods of ongoing conflict; explicit and diverse measures of youth exposure to political violence and armed conflict; and the examination of a wide range of process-oriented variables with the potential to inform theoretical models and translational intervention research. Tier 2 research thus importantly builds the pyramid of support for understanding and intervening in contexts of armed conflict by creating a rich pool of hypotheses about develop-mental processes that may be relevant to translational work. However, as a result of their cross-sectional designs, Tier 2 studies cannot provide definitive and ultimately reliable evidence for translation into intervention programs. Longitudinal, process-oriented research (e.g., Tier 3) is needed to follow up and specifically test the hypotheses laid out in Tier 2, in order to provide the strongest base for trans-lational work.

References

Al-Krenawi, A., Graham, J. R., & Kanat-Maymon, Y. (2009). Analysis of trauma exposure, symptomatology and functioning in Jewish Israeli and Palestinian adolescents. *British Journal of Psychiatry, 195*(5), 427–432. doi:10.1192/bjp.bp.108.050393.

Al-Krenawi, A., Slonim-Nevo, V., Maymon, Y., & Al-Krenawi, S. (2001). Psychological responses to blood vengeance among Arab adolescents. *Child Abuse and Neglect, 25*(4), 457–472. doi:10.1016/S0145-2134(01)00220-4.

Almqvist, K., & Broberg, A. G. (1999). Mental health and social adjustment in young refugee children 3½ years after their arrival in Sweden. *Journal of the American Academy of Child and Adolescent Psychiatry, 38*(6), 723–730. doi:10.1097/00004583-199906000-00020.

Barber, B. K. (1999). Political violence, family relations, and Palestinian youth functioning. *Journal of Adolescent Research, 14*(2), 206–230. doi:10.1177/0743558499142004.

Barber, B. K. (2001). Political violence, social integration, and youth functioning: Palestinian youth from the Intifada. *Journal of Community Psychology, 29*(3), 259–280. doi:10.1002/jcop.1017.

Betancourt, T. S., Brennan, R. T., Rubin-Smith, J., Fitzmaurice, G. M., & Gilman, S. E. (2010). Sierra Leone's former child soldiers: A longitudinal study of risk, protective factors, and mental health. *Journal of the American Academy of Child and Adolescent Psychiatry, 49*(6), 606–615. doi:10.1016/j.jaac.2010.03.008.

Betancourt, T. S., Salhi, C., Buka, S., Leaning, J., Dunn, G., & Earls, F. (2012). Connectedness, social support and internalising emotional and behavioural problems in adolescents displaced by the Chechen conflict. *Disasters, 36*(4), 635–655. doi:10.1111/j.1467-7717.2012.01280.x.

Bronfenbrenner, U. (1979). *The ecology of human development: Experiments by nature and design.* Cambridge, MA: Harvard University Press.

Bronfenbrenner, U. (1986). Ecology of the family as a context for human development: Research perspectives. *Developmental Psychology, 22*(6), 723–742. doi:10.1037/0012-1649.22.6.723.

Cummings, E. M., Goeke-Morey, M. C., Merrilees, C. E., Taylor, L. K., & Shirlow, P. (2014). A social-ecological, process-oriented perspective on political violence and child development. *Child Development Perspectives, 8*(2), 82–89. doi:10.1111/cdep.12067.

Dimitry, L. (2011). A systematic review on the mental health of children and adolescents in areas of armed conflict in the Middle East. *Child: Care, Health, and Development, 38*(2), 153–161. doi:10.1111/j.1365-2214.2011.01246.x.

Dubow, E. F., Boxer, P., Huesmann, L. R., Shikaki, K., Landau, S., Gvirsman, S. D., et al. (2010). Exposure to conflict and violence across contexts: Relations to adjustment across Palestinian children. *Journal of Clinical Child and Adolescent Psychology, 39*(1), 103–116. doi:10.1080/15374410903401153.

Duraković-Belko, E., Kulenović, A., & Đapić, R. (2003). Determinants of posttraumatic adjustment in adolescents from Sarajevo who experienced war. *Journal of Clinical Psychology, 59*(1), 27–40. doi:10.1002/jclp.10115.

Elbedour, S., ten Bensel, R., & Bastien, D. T. (1993). Ecological integrated model of children of war: Individual and social psychology. *Child Abuse and Neglect, 17*(6), 805–819.

Feldman, R., Vengrover, A., Eidelman-Rothman, M., & Zagoory-Sharon, O. (2013). Stress reactivity in war-exposed young children with and without posttraumatic stress disorder: relations to maternal stress hormones, parenting, and child emotionality and regulation. *Development and Psychopathology, 25*(4), 943–955. doi:10.1017/S0954579413000291.

Furr, J. M., Comer, J. S., Edmunds, J. M., & Kendall, P. C. (2010). Disasters and youth: A meta-analytic examination of posttraumatic stress. *Journal of Consulting and Clinical Psychology, 78*(6), 765–780. doi:10.1037/a0021482.

Harel-Fisch, Y., Radwan, Q., Walsh, S. D., Laufer, A., Amitai, G., Fogel-Grinvald, H., et al. (2010). Psychosocial outcomes related to subjective threat from armed conflict events (STACE): Findings from the Israeli-Palestinian cross-cultural HBSC study. *Child Abuse and Neglect, 34*(9), 623–638. doi:10.1016/j.chiabu.2009.12.007.

Jones, L., & Kafetsios, K. (2005). Exposure to political violence and psychological wellbeing in Bosnian adolescents: A mixed method approach. *Clinical Child Psychology and Psychiatry, 10* (2), 157–176. doi:10.1177/1359104505051209.

Joshi, P. T., & O'Donnell, D. A. (2003). Consequences of child exposure to war and terrorism. *Clinical Child and Family Psychology Review, 6*(4), 275–292. doi:10.1023/B:CCFP. 0000006294.88201.68.

Keresteš, G. (2006). Children's aggressive and prosocial behavior in relation to war exposure: Testing the role of perceived parenting and child's gender. *International Journal of Behavioral Development, 30*(3), 227–239. doi:10.1177/0165025406066756.

Khamis, V. (2012). Impact of war, religiosity and ideology on PTSD and psychiatric disorders in adolescents from Gaza Strip and South Lebanon. *Social Science and Medicine, 74*(12), 2005–2011. doi:10.1016/j.socscimed.2012.02.025.

Kohrt, B. A., Jordans, M. J. D., Tol, W. A., Perera, E., Karki, R., Koirala, S., et al. (2010). Social ecology of child soldiers: Child, family, and community determinants of mental health, psychosocial wellbeing, and reintegration in Nepal. *Transcultural Psychiatry, 47*(5), 727–753. doi:10.1177/1363461510381290.

Laor, N., Wolmer, L., Alon, M., Siev, J., Samuel, E., & Toren, P. (2006). Risk and protective factors mediating psychological symptoms and ideological commitment of adolescents facing continuous terrorism. *Journal of Nervous and Mental Disease, 194*(4), 279–286. doi:10.1097/01.nmd.0000207364.68064.dc.

Laor, N., Wolmer, L., & Cohen, D. J. (2001). Mothers' functioning and children's symptoms 5 years after a SCUD missile attack. *American Journal of Psychiatry, 158*(7), 1020–1026. doi:10.1176/appi.ajp.158.7.1020.

Laufer, A., Raz-Hamama, Y., Levine, S. Z., & Solomon, Z. (2009). Posttraumatic growth in adolescence: The role of religiosity, distress, and forgiveness. *Journal of Social and Clinical Psychology, 28*(7), 862–880. doi:10.1521/jscp.2009.28.7.862.

Laufer, A., & Solomon, Z. (2011). The role of religious orientations in youth's posttraumatic symptoms after exposure to terror. *Journal of Religion and Health, 50*(3), 687–699. doi:10.1007/s10943-009-9270-x.

Lavi, I., & Slone, M. (2011). Resilience and political violence: A cross-cultural study of moderating effects among Jewish and Arab-Israeli youth. *Youth & Society, 43*(3), 845–872. doi:10.1177/0044118X09353437.

Llabre, M. M., & Hadi, F. (1997). Social support and psychological distress in Kuwaiti boys and girls exposed to the Gulf Crisis. *Journal of Clinical Child Psychology, 26*(3), 247–255. doi:10.1207/s15374424jccp2603_3.

Merrilees, C. E., Cairns, E., Goeke-Morey, M., Schermerhorn, A. C., Shirlow, P., & Cummings, E. M. (2011). Associations between mothers' experience with the Troubles in Northern Ireland and mothers' and children's psychological functioning: The moderating role of social identity. *Journal of Community Psychology, 39*(1), 60–75. doi:doi:10.1002/jcop.20417.

Newnham, E. A., Pearson, R. M., Stein, A., & Betancourt, T. S. (2015). Youth mental health after civil war: The importance of daily stressors. *The British Journal of Psychiatry, 206,* 116–121.

O'Donnell, D. A., Schwab-Stone, M. E., & Muveed, A. Z. (2002). Multidimensional resilience in urban children exposed to community violence. *Child Development, 73*(4), 1265–1282. doi:10.1111/1467-8624.00471.

Panter-Brick, C., Eggerman, M., Gonzalez, V., & Safdar, S. (2009). Violence, suffering, and mental health in Afghanistan: A school-based survey. *Lancet, 374*(9692), 807–816. doi:10.1016/S0140-6736(09)61080-1.

Peltonen, K., Quota, S., El-Sarraj, E., & Punamäki, R.-L. (2010). Military trauma and social development: The moderating and mediating roles of peer and sibling relations in mental health. *International Journal of Behavioral Development, 34*(6), 554–563. doi:10.1177/0165025410368943.

Punamäki, R.-L., Muhammed, A. H., & Abdulrahman, H. A. (2004). Impact of traumatic events on coping strategies and their effectiveness among Kurdish children. *International Journal of Behavioral Development, 28*(1), 59–70. doi:10.1080/01650250344000271.

Punamäki, R.-L., & Puhakka, T. (1997). Determinants and effectiveness of children's coping with political violence. *International Journal of Behavioral Development, 21*(2), 349–370.

Punamäki, R.-L., Quota, S., & El-Sarraj, E. (2001). Resiliency factors predicting psychological adjustment after political violence among Palestinian children. *International Journal of Behavioral Development, 25*(3), 256–267. doi:10.1080/01650250042000294.

Qouta, S., Punamäki, R.-L., Miller, T., & E. l Sarraj, E. (2008). Does war beget child aggression? Military violence, gender, age and aggressive behavior in two Palestinian samples. *Aggressive Behavior, 34*(3), 231–244. doi:10.1002/ab/20236.

Sagy, S. (2006). Hope in times of threat: The case of Palestinian and Israeli-Jewish youth. *American Journal of Orthopsychiatry, 76*(1), 128–133.

Schiff, M. (2006). Living in the shadow of terrorism: Psychological distress and alcohol use among religious and non-religious adolescents in Jerusalem. *Social Science and Medicine, 62* (9), 2301–2312. doi:10.1016/j.socscimed.2005.10.016.

Shahar, G., Cohen, G., Grogan, K. E., Barile, J. P., & Henrich, C. C. (2009). Terrorism-related perceived stress, adolescent depression, and social support from friends. *Pediatrics, 124*(2), E235–E240. doi:10.1542/peds.2008-2971.

Slone, M., Lobel, T., & Gilat, I. (1999). Dimensions of the political environment affecting children's mental health: An Israeli study. *The Journal of Conflict Resolution, 43*(1), 78–91. doi:10.1177/0022002799043001005.

Smith, P., Perrin, S., Yule, W., & Rabe-Hesketh, S. (2001). War exposure and maternal reactions in the psychological adjustment of children from Bosnia-Hercegovina. *Journal of Child Psychology and Psychiatry and Allied Disciplines, 42*(3), 395–404. doi:10.1017/S002196300100765.

Thabet, A. A., Ibraheem, A. N., Shivram, R., Winter, E. A., & Vostanis, P. (2009). Parenting support and PTSD in children of a war zone. *International Journal of Social Psychiatry, 55*(3), 226–237. doi:10.1177/0020764008096100.

Tol, W. A., Song, S. Z., & Jordans, J. D. (2013). Annual research review: Resilience and mental health in children and adolescents living in areas of armed conflict—a systematic review of findings in low- and middle-income countries. *Journal of Child Psychology and Psychiatry, 54* (4), 445–460. doi:10.1111/jcpp.12053.

Ungar, M. (2015). Practitioner review: Diagnosing childhood resilience—a systemic approach to the diagnosis of adaptation in adverse social and physical ecologies. *Journal of Child Psychology and Psychiatry, 56*(1), 4–17. doi:10.1111/jcpp.12306.

Chapter 6
Tier 3: Longitudinal Studies of Mediators, Moderators, and Multiple Social-Ecological Levels

Keywords Longitudinal mediation · Emotional security theory · Family violence and support · Community violence and acceptance · Within-person change

Tier 3 research, as we define it, expands beyond Tier 2 by *prospectively* exploring pre-, mid-, and/or postconflict factors that mediate and moderate the effects of exposure to political violence and armed conflict on youth adjustment in multiple contexts (see Fig. 3.1). As in Tier 2, Tier 3 includes exploration of psychological and social variables. In the course of our review, we identified 25 studies that fit the criteria for Tier 3. In this section, we will discuss noteworthy findings and patterns from this body of work. For the sake of consistency with the other tiers, we also selected a diverse subset of Tier 3 studies ($N = 20$) using the previously discussed criteria and have presented them in detail in Table 6.1. Notably, as with previous Table 6.1 should not be regarded as a comprehensive listing of all Tier 3 studies that exist in the empirical literature. The aim of this table is to present a representative sample of diverse and exemplary work conducted at the Tier 3 level.

A Process-Oriented, Social-Ecological Perspective

Tier 3 research generally reflects process-oriented, social-ecological perspectives on youth adjustment in contexts of political violence. Whereas the primary contributions of Tiers 1 and 2 research have been to build up a knowledge base about cross-sectional correlations between exposure to political violence and youth adjustment, Tier 3 provides longitudinal evidence of the dynamic processes that account for negative or positive outcomes. *Dynamic processes* refer to the particular and often complex organizations of cognitive, socio-emotional, physiological and other processes that reflect youths' functioning over time in particular contexts, including bidirectional and multiple forms of change (e.g., Cummings & Valentino, 2015).

Critically, Tier 3 research accounts for the transactions of person and process in terms of the effects of histories and development over time. In other words, Tier 3

© Springer International Publishing AG 2017
E.M. Cummings et al., *Political Violence, Armed Conflict, and Youth Adjustment*,
DOI 10.1007/978-3-319-51583-0_6

studies search for more than just markers of risk, but also for characterizations of how and why psychological, physiological, and other factors interactively influence child development. Testing well-articulated theoretical models provides an informative assessment of the possible processes underlying developmental change. Such tests are typically based on structural equation modeling (SEM) and optimally require at least three waves of data collection so that predictors, mediators, and outcomes are assessed at different points in time (Maxwell & Cole, 2007). However, albeit offering specific advantages for identifying mediating processes as causal agents (Cole & Maxwell, 2003), SEM model tests typically between-person analyses, which leaves questions about explanatory processes as mechanisms of change over time from a person-oriented (e.g., within-person) perspective (Sterba & Bauer, 2010). It is also informative to characterize pathways due to exposure to political violence in terms of casual processes occurring at the within-person level —for example, the processes that account for person-oriented continuity and change in adaptation and maladaptation over time (Bergman, von Eye, & Magnusson, 2006; Cummings & Valentino, 2015). Accordingly, in addition to testing theoretical models, many Tier 3 studies examine the ontogeny of individual trajectories of development over time (Cummings, Davies, & Campbell, 2000).

We will now discuss key findings and patterns from Tier 3, organized by levels of the social ecology. Given that studies in Tier 3 often included multiple characteristics described above, we will describe studies as exemplars for the given level of the social ecology and then present studies that have incorporated multiple levels of the social ecology and those that have examined within-person change.

Individual characteristics A variety of individual characteristics, including psychological processes, have been examined in the Tier 3 literature. For example, in a two-year study of former child soldiers in Sierra Leone, Betancourt and colleagues (2010) reported that young rape survivors exhibited increases in anxiety, hostility, confidence, and prosocial behavior across time-points, whereas youth who had wounded or killed others exhibited increases in hostility. Another study examined PTSD symptoms in the context of the war in Croatia, with assessments during and after the war (Kuterovac-Jagodić, 2003). The authors reported that, despite significant declines in symptoms over time, 10% of children continued to report severe levels of symptoms 30 months postwar.

Regulatory processes are another important subset of individual processes that have been assessed for youth in contexts of political violence and armed conflict. For example, emotional insecurity has been repeatedly associated with youth adjustment over time in contexts of political violence (e.g., Bar-Tal & Jacobson, 1998; Batniji, Rabaia, Nguyen-Gillham, Giacaman, Sarraj, Punamäki, Saab, & Boyce, 2009; Hobfoll, Hall, Canetti-Nisim, Galea, Johnson, & Palmieri, 2007; McAloney, McCrystal, Percy, & McCarttan, 2009); emotional security theory (Davies et al., 1994) has roots in attachment theory (Bowlby, 1969, 1973) and posits that youth adjustment is influenced by the quality of the larger social ecology (e.g., community, culture, and political context). Studies by Cummings and colleagues have shown with both between- and within-person tests that emotional

Table 6.1 Tier 3

Region and conflict	Reference	Sample	Assessment timing	Measures	Major findings
Africa					
Burundi; ongoing conflict between the Hutu and Tutsi ethnic groups	Hall, Tol, Jordans, Bass, and de Jong (2014)	• 176 youth (*M* age at baseline = 12 years) who had been exposed to one or more potentially traumatic life events and who exhibited significant levels of psychological distress at baseline	• Three assessments across 4 months • Peace agreements were signed three years before T1, but threats of violence persisted	• Depression • PTSD • Functional impairment • Received social support • Cognitive social capital (youth trust, cohesion, and reciprocity in the community)	• Higher levels of cognitive social capital were associated with reductions in both depressive symptoms and functional impairment between T1 and T2, and between T2 and T3 • Higher levels of cognitive social capital were positively associated with increases in social support between T1 and T2 and T2 and T3
Sierra Leone; Sierra Leone Civil War	Betancourt, Agnew-Blais, Gilman, Williams, and Ellis (2010a)	• 152 former child soldiers (*M* age at T2 = 17.39 years) who had been served by Interim Care Centers	• Two assessments, 2 years apart • T1 data collection occurred the year the war ended	• War experiences • Psychological adjustment • Perceived discrimination • Family acceptance • School retention • Community acceptance	• Postconflict discrimination explained a large proportion of the relationship between past experiences of hurting or killing others and later increases in hostility • Postconflict discrimination was inversely associated with both family and community acceptance • Higher levels of baseline community acceptance and increases in community acceptance between time-points were related to higher levels of adaptive

(continued)

Table 6.1 (continued)

Region and conflict	Reference	Sample	Assessment timing	Measures	Major findings
					behaviors and attitudes over time • Increases in family acceptance between time-points were inversely associated with hostility at T2 • Stigma positively mediated the relationship between rape survival and depression • Rape survival was independently associated with increases in hostility, anxiety, and prosocial behaviors
Sierra Leone; Sierra Leone Civil War	Betancourt, Brennan, Rubin-Smith, Fitzmaurice, and Gilman (2010b)	• 260 former child soldiers (M age at T1 = 15.13 years) who had been served by Interim Care Centers	• Three assessments, 2 and 4 years apart • T1 data collection occurred the year the war ended	• War experiences • Psychosocial adjustment • Perceived support • Daily hardships • Perceived discrimination	• Rape survivors exhibited higher levels of internalizing problems at T1 than those who had not been raped • School attendance and higher levels of community acceptance were positively associated with prosocial/adaptive behaviors at T1 • Increases in community acceptance were associated with decreased internalizing and externalizing problems over time • Social and economic hardships and younger age at the time of

(continued)

Table 6.1 (continued)

Region and conflict	Reference	Sample	Assessment timing	Measures	Major findings
					• involvement with fighting forces were positively associated with increases in internalizing problems over time • Postconflict stigma and histories of injuring or killing others were positively associated with decreases in prosocial/adaptive behaviors over time • Social support and increases in community acceptance were associated with increases in prosocial/adaptive behaviors over time
Sierra Leone; Sierra Leone Civil War	Betancourt et al. (2010b)	• 156 former child soldiers (*M* age at T1 = 15.13 years) who had been served by Interim Care Centers	• Two assessments, 2 years apart • T1 data collection occurred the year the war ended	• War experiences • Psychosocial adjustment • Family acceptance • School retention • Community acceptance	• Rape survivors exhibited higher levels of anxiety, as well as greater confidence and prosocial attitudes at T2 than T1 • Rape survivors and those who had perpetrated killing exhibited significantly higher hostility at T2 than T1 • Improvements in community acceptance between time-points were associated with reductions in depressive symptoms, improved

(continued)

Table 6.1 (continued)

Region and conflict	Reference	Sample	Assessment timing	Measures	Major findings
					confidence, and improved prosocial attitudes at T2, above and beyond levels of exposure to violence
Sierra Leone; Civil War	Betancourt, McBain, Newnham, and Brennan (2013)	• 529 youth (M age at T1 = 14.48 years), including former child soldiers who had been served by Interim Care Centers ($n = 264$), war-affected youth who had not been served by Centers ($n = 137$), and a cohort of self-reintegrated former child soldiers who were recruited at T2 ($n = 127$)	• Three assessments, 2 and 4 years apart • T1 data collection occurred the year the war ended	• War experiences • Psychological problems • Social disorder • Daily hardships • Functional impairment • Risky behavior • Perceived stigma • Intergenerational closure • Community acceptance	• Despite very limited access to care, the majority of participants maintained low levels of internalizing problems or exhibited significant improvements over time • A minority of the sample maintained severe internalizing symptoms or reported worsened symptoms at T3, compared to T1 and T2 • Caregiver loss, family abuse and neglect, and community stigma were positively associated with ongoing internalizing problems over time
Sierra Leone; Sierra Leone Civil War	Betancourt, McBain, Newnham, and Brennan (2014)	• 243 former child soldiers (M age at baseline of present study = 16.6 years) and caregivers who participated in a larger prospective study • The sample included youth who received reintegration	• Larger study involved three assessments, conducted 2 and 4 years apart • Present study used data from T2 and T3 of the	• War experiences (youth report) • Youth mental health (youth report) • Daily hardships (youth report)	• Higher levels of community social disorder were positively associated with internalizing and externalizing problems at both baseline and follow-up

(continued)

Table 6.1 (continued)

Region and conflict	Reference	Sample	Assessment timing	Measures	Major findings
		services ($n = 127$) and youth who self-reintegrated ($n = 116$)	larger study (conducted 4 years apart) • Present study's data collection occurred 2 and 6 years postwar, respectively	• Family abuse/acceptance (youth report) • Community collective efficacy (caregiver report) • Community social disorder (caregiver report) • Perceived stigma by the community (youth report)	• Higher levels of perceived stigma by the community were positively associated with internalizing and externalizing problems at both baseline and follow-up • Several gender differences in predictors and trajectories of internalizing and externalizing problems emerged • Collective efficacy was not significantly associated with internalizing or externalizing problems
Sierra Leone; Sierra Leone Civil War	Betancourt, McBain, Newnham, and Brennan (2015)	• 118 former child soldiers (M age at baseline of the present study = 16.5 years) and caregivers who participated in a larger prospective study • The sample included youth who had received reintegration services from a non-government agency, youth who had not received reintegration services, and self-reintegrated youth	• Larger study involved three assessments, conducted two and four years apart • Present study used data from T2 and T3 of the larger study (conducted four years apart) • Present study's data collection occurred 2 and 6 years postwar, respectively	• War experiences (youth report) • Youth internalizing symptoms (youth report) • Caregiver internalizing symptoms (caregiver report) • Family acceptance (youth report) • Daily hardships • Community stigma (youth report)	• Changes in caregiver anxiety/depression between time-points were positively and robustly associated with changes in youth internalizing symptoms • Increases in family acceptance between time-points were positively associated with improvements in youth internalizing symptoms • Reductions in community stigma between time-points were positively associated

(continued)

Table 6.1 (continued)

Region and conflict	Reference	Sample	Assessment timing	Measures	Major findings
					with improvements in youth internalizing symptoms
Sierra Leone; Sierra Leone Civil War	Betancourt, Newnham, McBain, and Brennan (2013)	• 243 former child soldiers (M age at baseline = 16.6 years), including former child soldiers who had been served by Interim Care Centers (n = 127) and self-reintegrated former child soldiers (n = 116)	• Three assessments, 2 and 4 years apart • T1 data collection occurred the year the war ended	• War experiences • PTSD • Perceived stigma • Family acceptance • Family abuse and neglect • School participation • Services received after the war	• Despite limited access to psychological care, approximately one-third of participants reported improvements in PTSD symptoms between T1 and T3 • Females reported higher levels of PTSD at baseline than males; however, gender differences were not evident at follow-up • Parental death and increases in community stigma were associated with worsening PTSD symptoms over time • Increases in family acceptance were associated with improvements in PTSD symptoms over time
Uganda; Lord's Resistance Army insurgency	Haroz et al. (2013)	• 102 Acholi youth (M age = 15 years) living in internal displacement person camps	• Two assessments, six months apart • Data collection occurred in IDP camps during a period of ongoing conflict	• Adverse life events • Psychological symptoms • Prosocial behaviors • Perceived social support	• High levels of prosocial behavior at T1 were associated with improvements in anxiety symptoms among participants who exhibited high symptom improvement • Recent caregiver loss moderated modified the

(continued)

Table 6.1 (continued)

Region and conflict	Reference	Sample	Assessment timing	Measures	Major findings
					relationship between prosocial behavior at T1 and depressive trajectories. When comparing youth with high versus low prosocial behaviors, those who did not experience caregiver loss reported greater improvements in depressive symptoms than those who did lose caregivers • Social support at T1 was not significantly associated with reductions in anxiety or depressive symptoms over time
Asia					
Afghanistan; ongoing political violence and armed conflict	Panter-Brick, Goodman, Tol, and Eggerman (2011)	• 234 child–caregiver dyads (*M* youth age at baseline= 13.5 years) that completed repeated measures of a larger school-based mental health survey	• Two assessments, 1 year apart • Data collection occurred during a period of ongoing conflict	• Youth exposure to traumatic events • Youth psychological symptoms • Youth PTSD • Caregiver psychological symptoms • Stressors • Protective factors	• Youth psychological symptoms improved significantly between time-points, with the exception of PTSD • Greater cumulative life trauma was associated with higher levels of PTSD symptoms • Higher levels of family violence prospectively predicted worsening non-PTSD symptoms between T1 and T2

(continued)

Table 6.1 (continued)

Region and conflict	Reference	Sample	Assessment timing	Measures	Major findings
					• Higher levels of major family conflict prospectively predicted worsening depressive symptoms between T1 and T2 • Improvements in family life between T1 and T2 were associated with better youth mental health outcomes at T2
Palestine; Gaza War	Palosaari, Punamäki, Diab, and Qouta (2013)	• 240 youth (M age = 11.35 years)	• Three assessments, 2 and 6 months apart • Data collection three, five, and 11 months after the war, respectively	• War trauma • Peri-traumatic dissociation • PTSD • Post-traumatic cognitions	• Peri-traumatic cognition levels predicted later levels and changes in PTSD symptoms •PTSD symptom levels did not predict peri-traumatic cognitions over time • Changes in PTSD symptoms did not predict peri-traumatic cognitions over time • There was no evidence that baseline PTSD symptoms developed into chronic symptoms via negative peri-traumatic cognitions
Palestine; Gaza War	Boxer et al. (2013)	• 1,501 youth from three age cohorts (8, 11, and 14 years) and their parents The youth sample included Palestinians (n = 600), Israeli Jews (n = 451) and Arab Israelis (n = 450.)	• Three annual assessments • Data collection occurred during a period of ongoing conflict, several years after the Second Intifada	• Youth exposure to ethnic-political conflict and violence (parent report for 8-year-olds, youth report for 11- and 14-year-olds) Youth exposure to school conflict and violence (youth report) Youth exposure to family	• Exposure to ethno-political violence at T1 was positively associated with microsystem (e.g., family, school, community) violence at T2 for all age cohorts • Exposure to microsystem violence at T2 predicted

(continued)

Table 6.1 (continued)

Region and conflict	Reference	Sample	Assessment timing	Measures	Major findings
				conflict and violence (youth report) Youth aggressive behavior (youth and parent reports)	increases in aggression across time-points among the youngest age cohort • Exposure to ethno-political violence at T2 was positively associated with aggression at T3 among all age cohorts
Palestine and Israel; ongoing Israeli Palestinian conflict	Dubow et al. (2012)	• 1,501 youth from three age cohorts (8, 11, and 14 years) and their parents • The youth sample included Palestinians (*n* = 600), Israeli Jews (*n* = 451), and Arab Israelis (*n* = 450)	• Three annual assessments • Data collection occurred during a period of ongoing conflict, several years after the Second Intifada	• Youth exposure to ethnic-political conflict and violence (parent report for 8-year-olds, youth report for 11- and 14-year-olds) • Youth PTSD (youth report) • Youth self-esteem (youth report) • Youth academic grades (parent report) • Parent mental health (parent report) • Positive parenting (parent report)	• Greater cumulative exposure to ethnic-political conflict/violence across T1 and T2 predicted higher levels of PTSD symptoms at subsequent time-points, above and beyond initial symptom levels • Youth self-esteem moderated the relationship between cumulative exposure and PTSD symptoms. Youth who had been exposed to higher levels of ethnic-political conflict/violence and who reported lower levels of self-esteem were more likely to report PTSD symptoms at T3 • Positive parenting moderated the relationship between cumulative exposure and

(continued)

Table 6.1 (continued)

Region and conflict	Reference	Sample	Assessment timing	Measures	Major findings
					PTSD symptoms. Youth who had been exposed to high levels of ethnic-political conflict/violence and who reported low levels of positive parenting were more likely to report PTSD symptoms at T3
Europe					
Croatia; Croatian War of Independence	Kuterovac-Jagodić (2003)	• 252 youth (*M* age at baseline = 10.83 years) from a town exposed to massive military attacks	• Two assessments, 3 years apart. • T1 data collection occurred mid-war. • T2 data collection occurred 30 months after the war ended	• War experiences • PTSD • Externality of control • Coping strategies • Perceived social support	• Most participants' PTSD symptoms declined over time; however, many participants still exhibited high symptom levels at follow-up • War exposure intensity, separation from family members, and displacement positively predicted short-term, but not long-term, PTSD symptoms • PTSD symptom intensity at T1 strongly and positively predicted long-term symptoms • Coping strategies and locus of control predicted long-term, but not short-term, PTSD symptoms. The exception was emotional coping strategies, which predicted short-term symptoms

(continued)

Table 6.1 (continued)

Region and conflict	Reference	Sample	Assessment timing	Measures	Major findings
					• Aggressive coping strategies were associated with high levels of long-term PTSD symptoms • Higher levels of social support were associated with lower levels of long-term PTSD symptoms
Ireland; the Troubles	Cummings et al. (2011)	• 695 mother–child dyads (M youth age at baseline = 12.17 years) from economically deprived Belfast neighborhoods	• Three annual assessments • Data collection occurred several years after formal peace accords, but during a period of ongoing ethnic segregation and community violence	• Youth exposure to sectarian and nonsectarian community violence (youth report) • Youth adjustment problems (youth and mother reports) • Youth aggression (youth report) • Youth insecurity about the community (mother report)	• Sectarian community violence exerted longitudinal effects on youths' internalizing and externalizing symptoms, mediated by heightened emotional insecurity about the community, controlling for T1 internalizing and externalizing symptoms • Nonsectarian community violence was directly and positively associated with youth's internalizing problems at T3, controlling for T1 internalizing symptoms • Relations between politically driven community violence and youth's internalizing problems were stronger for younger than older children

(continued)

Table 6.1 (continued)

Region and conflict	Reference	Sample	Assessment timing	Measures	Major findings
Ireland; the Troubles	Cummings et al. (2012)	• 299 mother–child dyads (*M* youth age at baseline = 12.33 years) from two-parent families (married or living as married) from economically deprived Belfast neighborhoods	• Three annual assessments • Data collection occurred several years after formal peace accords, but during a period of ongoing ethnic segregation and community violence	• Historical political violence (e.g., death rates) • Youth exposure to sectarian and nonsectarian community violence (youth report) • Youth adjustment problems (youth and mother reports) • Youth emotional insecurity about the family (youth and mother reports) • Family conflict (mother report)	• Family conflict and youths' insecurity about family relationships emerged as mechanisms underlying the relationship between historical political violence, sectarian antisocial behavior, and youth's adjustment problems • Family conflict and youths' insecurity about family relationships emerged as mechanisms mediating the relationship between sectarian antisocial behavior and youths' internalizing and externalizing problems at T3, controlling for T1 internalizing and externalizing problems
Ireland; the Troubles	Cummings, Merrilees, Taylor, Shirlow, Goeke-Morey, and Cairns (2013a).	• 1,015 mother–child dyads (*M* youth age at baseline = 12.14 years) from economically deprived Belfast neighborhoods	• Four annual assessments. • Data collection occurred several years after formal peace accords, but during a period of ongoing ethnic segregation community violence	• Police records of crime • Youth exposure to sectarian and nonsectarian community violence (youth report) • Youth total adjustment problems (youth and mother reports)	• Exposure to sectarian community violence predicted higher levels of long-term youth total adjustment problems • Neighborhood crime rates moderated these relations; relations between sectarian community violence and

(continued)

Table 6.1 (continued)

Region and conflict	Reference	Sample	Assessment timing	Measures	Major findings
					increased youth adjustment problems were accentuated in high-crime neighborhoods
Ireland; the Troubles	Cummings, Taylor, Merrilees, Goeke-Morey, Shirlow, and Cairns (2013b)	• 999 mother–child dyads (M youth age at baseline = 12.19 years) from economically deprived Belfast neighborhoods	• Four annual assessments • Data collection occurred several years after formal peace accords, but during a period of ongoing ethnic segregation and community violence	• Youth exposure to sectarian community violence (youth report) • Youth conduct problems (youth and mother reports) • Youth emotion problems (youth and mother reports) • Youth emotional insecurity about the community (mother report)	• Youth's trajectories of greater emotional insecurity over four waves of assessment were positively related to risk for developing conduct and emotional problems, respectively • Analyses took into account earlier adjustment problems, age, and gender, and the time-varying nature of sectarian violence over the four waves of assessment recovery across waves significantly predicted the development of conduct and emotional problems
Ireland; the Troubles	Merrilees, Cairns, Taylor, Goeke-Morey, Shirlow, Cummings (2013)	• 770 mother–child dyads (M youth age at baseline = 13.58 years) from economically deprived Belfast neighborhoods	• Two annual assessments • Data collection occurred several years after formal peace accords, but during a period of ongoing ethnic segregation and community violence	• Youth exposure to sectarian and nonsectarian community violence (youth report) • Youth social identity (youth report) • Youth aggression (youth report) • Youth delinquency (youth report)	• Exposure to sectarian antisocial behavior was significantly associated with increases in general and sectarian aggression and delinquency between time-points • In-group social identity moderated the impact of

(continued)

Table 6.1 (continued)

Region and conflict	Reference	Sample	Assessment timing	Measures	Major findings
				• Youth conduct problems (mother report) • Youth sectarian aggression (youth report)	sectarian community violence on youth adjustment problems, strengthening relations with aggression and delinquency toward the out-group relations and weakening relations with general aggressive behavior • The relations between sectarian community violence and sectarian aggression were stronger for males than females
Ireland; the Troubles	Merrilees et al. (2014b)	• 814 youth (M age at the present study's baseline = 13.61 years) from economically deprived Belfast neighborhoods who participated in at least one of the third, fourth, or fifth waves of a larger prospective study	• Three annual assessments • Data collection occurred several years after formal peace accords, but during a period of ongoing ethnic and community violence	• Youth exposure to sectarian community violence • Youth emotional problems • Youth group identity strength	• The relationship between sectarian community violence and youth's emotional problems was stronger among older than younger adolescents • Youth who reported higher group identity strength reported significantly fewer emotional problems in contexts of sectarian community violence. This effect was more pronounced among Protestants than Catholics

security mediates the impact of political violence and adjustment problems. More specifically, youth exposed to higher levels of political violence report higher levels of emotional insecurity which in turn related to higher levels of internalizing and externalizing symptoms (e.g., Cummings et al., 2011, 2012; Cummings, Merrilees, Taylor, Shirlow, Goeke-Morey, & Cairns, 2013a; Cummings, Taylor, Merrilees, Goeke-Morey, & Shirlow, 2013b). Interrelations between emotional insecurity about family and community in relating to youth adjustment were found based on five-wave tests of trajectories of emotional insecurity (Cummings et al., 2016). Greater insecurity about the community exacerbated the negative impact of family conflict on insecurity about the family, suggesting that insecurity about the community sensitizes youth to family conflict. Youth's religiosity (Goeke-Morey, Taylor, Merrilees, Shirlow, & Cummings, 2014), group identity, and interrelations between youth's group identity and emotional insecurity (Merrilees, Goeke-Morey, Shirlow, and Cummings 2014a, 2014b) were also identified as individual characteristics related to youth's adjustment and development over time.

Rigorous tests of other specific psychological processes have also begun to emerge in the Tier 3 literature. For example, in a three-wave study of PTSD symptoms among Palestinian children in the aftermath of the 2008 Israeli Palestinian conflict, Palosaari, Punamäki, Diab, and Qouta (2013) reported that peri-traumatic cognitions predicted later levels and changes in PTSD symptoms; however, they found no evidence that baseline PTSD symptoms developed into chronic symptoms over time through negative peri-traumatic cognitions.

Microsystem factors Family-level factors have repeatedly been identified as salient predictors of youth outcomes in Tier 3 studies. For example, in a one-year follow-up study of youth mental health in Afghanistan, Panter-Brick, Goodman, Tol, and Eggerman (2011) reported that family violence significantly predicted non-PTSD mental health symptoms, but that only lifetime trauma significantly predicted PTSD. These results demonstrate the importance of identifying specific sources of adversity in the social ecology that predict specific youth outcomes. Meanwhile, examining three waves of data from Sierra Leone, Betancourt, McBain, Newnham, and Brennan (2013) reported that caregiver loss and family abuse and neglect were positively associated with ongoing internalizing problems over time among war-affected youth, with postaccord family abuse linked to PTSD and higher levels of family acceptance linked to positive adjustment. In another three-wave test in Northern Ireland, Cummings and colleagues (2012) identified family conflict as part of a mediational chain linking exposure to sectarian antisocial behavior with youth internalizing and externalizing problems, with youth emotional security about family conflict acting as an even more proximal mediator of adjustment. Finally, Taylor, Merrilees, Goeke-Morey, Shirlow, and Cummings (2014) recently reported that family cohesion buffered the relationship between exposure to sectarian community violence and youth aggression in Northern Ireland.

Community-level factors have also been identified as important predictors of youth outcomes in Tier 3 studies. For example, in a two-wave growth model analysis of former child soldiers in Sierra Leone, Betancourt et al. (2014) reported that baseline, postconflict community characteristics (social disorder in the community, social stigma) predicted youth internalizing and externalizing problems at baseline and a four-year follow-up. In a prior two-wave analysis in Sierra Leone, Betancourt, Agnew-Blais, Gilman, Williams, and Ellis (2010a) also called attention to the influence of postwar social stigma on the psychological adjustment of former child soldiers and young rape survivors—reporting, for example, that postaccord discrimination explained a large proportion of the relationship between past experiences of hurting or killing others and later increases in hostility. Finally, in another study with former child soldiers in Sierra Leone, Betancourt and colleagues (2010c) reported that improvements in community acceptance over a two-year period were linked with increased prosocial attitudes, increased confidence, and reduced depressive symptoms.

Youth perceptions about community-level resources and threats may also exert direct and mediated influences on later adjustment. For example, Hall, Tol, Jordans, Bass, and de Jong (2014) examined related community dimensions in a three-wave study of Burundi children conducted over a period of 4 months. Using cross-lagged path analyses, they reported that high levels of social capital in the community (reflecting the extent to which youth believed their communities were cohesive and trustworthy) were linked to lower rates of depression and functional impairment, declining levels of mental health symptoms, and increased social support over time. Meanwhile, Cummings and colleagues (2011) analyzed three waves of data from Northern Ireland and reported that sectarian community violence was part of a mediational chain linked to youth internalizing and externalizing problems, with youths' emotional insecurity about community violence acting as a proximal mediator of adjustment. These two studies demonstrate how community-level processes may confer risk or protection for youth over time.

Beyond the microsystem Studies examining specific variables occurring at higher-order levels of the social ecology have been rare thus far; however, this is an important area for future work. In a notable example, Cummings and colleagues (2012) linked historical political violence in Northern Ireland, as indexed by a database drawn from police and other independent sources, with sectarian and nonsectarian community violence, as well as a chain of relations over time leading to youth internalizing and externalizing problems. Specifically, community histories of politically motivated deaths were found to be related to increased rates of both sectarian and nonsectarian community violence. Sectarian community violence was, in turn, shown to be related to higher levels of family conflict, which predicted youth's emotional insecurity. Emotional insecurity, in turn, was positively related to youth internalizing and externalizing problems. Similarly, Cummings and colleagues (2013a) prospectively examined community-level effects on youth adjustment in Northern Ireland across four waves, using three-level modeling that allowed for nesting of relations by neighborhood. They reported that exposure to sectarian antisocial behavior in the community predicted youth adjustment problems, a relationship that was elevated in higher crime neighborhoods.

Multiple levels of the social ecology Several Tier 3 studies have systematically and simultaneously examined multiple levels of the social ecology related to youth adjustment. For example, Boxer, Huesmann, Dubow, Landau, Gvirsman, Shikaki, & Ginges (2013) employed a three-wave test to examine the impact of multiple ecologies of violence on youth aggression in a diverse sample of Israeli Jews, Israeli Arabs, and Palestinians. They reported that baseline exposure to ethno-political violence was associated with increases in aggression between T2 and T3 by increasing school, family, and community violence between T1 and T2. Meanwhile, in another three-wave test, Dubow et al. (2010) reported that Palestinian children were at heightened risk for exposure to violence across multiple contexts compared to Israeli Jewish and Israeli Arab children. They also identified unique effects of exposure to violence in different contexts (ethno-political, family, school) at T1 and T2 on PTSD symptoms at T3, controlling for PTSD symptoms in the T1 and T2.

Within-person change and person-oriented analyses Several Tier 3 studies have also significantly contributed to knowledge by exploring between-person differences in within-person change over time. For example, analyzing youth emotional insecurity as a psychological process across multiple time-points in Northern Ireland, Cummings and colleagues (2013b) showed that within-person trajectories of emotional insecurity about the community were related to risk for emotion and conduct problems, including controls for earlier adjustment problems and youths' time-varying experiences with sectarian community violence (see also Cummings, Merrilees, Taylor, Goeke-Morey, & Shirlow, in press). In most prior research on emotional insecurity, emotional insecurity measured was assessed at a single point in time in the context of model testing using structural equation modeling (SEM). Thus, a particular advance of Cummings, Taylor, and colleagues' work was their demonstration of the psychological significance of developmental trajectories of emotional insecurity about the community, as measured at multiple time-points. In another study in Northern Ireland, Merrilees and colleagues (2014a) integrated emotional security theory and social identity theory to study youth adjustment over time. They reported that social identity and emotional security were longitudinally interrelated in adolescence and that differences in these relations were functions of specific ethno-political identities (e.g., Catholic, Protestant).

Finally, in a five-wave study in Northern Ireland, Cummings, Taylor, Merrilees, Goeke-Morey, & Shirlow (2016) employed hierarchical linear modeling (HLM) to model between-person differences in within-person change over time. They reported that within-person trajectories of emotional insecurity about the family were related to youth delinquency, with insecurity about the community increasing the negative impact of family conflict on youth insecurity about the family. These findings suggest that youth insecurity about the community sensitizes them to exposure to family conflict in the home, thus demonstrating the dynamic relations between youth insecurity about multiple levels of the social ecology. In another study examining between-person differences in within-person change over time, Punamäki et al. (2015) reported a three-trajectory solution of PTSD symptoms among Palestinian children who were assessed 3, 5, and 11 months postwar. They reported that, while 76% of their sample exhibited a recovery trajectory, the rest exhibited resistant or increasing symptoms trajectories. Youth membership in different trajectory classes was associated with both individual- and family-level factors.

Summary

Tier 3 studies examine adaptive and maladaptive processes of socio-emotional and cognitive functioning, as well as psychopathology outcomes. They also tease apart contextual influences, analyzing both positive and negative influences, processes, and outcomes (e.g., resilience). This work reflects an emerging consensus that the effects of political violence and armed conflict on youth are informatively conceptualized in terms of both direct effects on the individual, and in terms of the impact on individuals, families, communities, and other contexts in which youth live, including the psychological processes that these social ecologies influence and the factors that moderate outcomes. The longitudinal research designs employed in Tier 3 studies allow for advancements in the study of these factors, such as clarifying the directional relations over time between social ecologies of political violence, mediating psychological processes, and youth adjustment. These designs also allow for the study of change at multiple levels of the social ecology.

Table 6.1 documents in rich detail the approaches and regions of the world studied at the Tier 3 level, including tests of mediators, psychologically based moderators, levels of the social ecology, and other possible risk and protective factors for the impact of political violence on children from a process-oriented, longitudinal, social-ecological perspective. The research shows that multiple levels of the social ecology that are more proximal to youths' daily functioning than political violence and armed conflict are related to youth outcomes, including community and family functioning. These findings regarding risk and protective factors have implications for intervention research, specifically, suggesting that process-oriented intervention at the levels of the family and community may hold promise for ameliorating youth adjustment in the face of ethno-political violence (e.g., Boxer et al. 2013; Dubow et al. 2012). Relatedly, these findings suggest the promise of family and community intervention approaches by longitudinally supporting specific processes and contexts that could be targeted in the course of intervention. For example, the body of research by Betancourt, Borisova, and colleagues indicates that community and family acceptance, social support, and school attendance are protective factors for youth psychological well-being, whereas community stigma, histories of injuring or killing others, social and economic hardship, and caregiver loss and family abuse are risk factors. Studies by Cummings and colleagues support the role of community and family factors as mediators of youth adjustment, with historical political violence, politically driven community violence, neighborhood crime, and family conflict as risk factors.

Emotional security about the community, family, and parent–child relations is identified as acting as risk or protective processes, depending on whether relations are insecure or secure, respectively. Theoretical models based on emotional security and/or social identity theories (see Merrilees et al., 2014b) have received repeated support in three-, four-, and/or five-wave studies of youth adjustment and development in contexts of political violence in Northern Ireland (see review in Cummings et al. 2014; 2016), providing longitudinal, process-oriented bases for theoretical models about risk and protective factors to potentially guide translational research studies.

Despite the promise of Tier 3 research, our review revealed a paucity of research laboratories engaged in Tier 3 research (see Table 6.1), reflecting the need for exploration of these issues by many more research groups in many more contexts, with the goal of optimally informing future translational research.

References

Bar-Tal, D., & Jacobson, D. (1998). A psychological perspective on security. *Applied Psychology: An International Review, 47*(1), 59–71. doi:10.1080/0269999498378079.

Batniji, R., Rabaia, Y., Nguyen-Gillham, V., Giacaman, R., Sarraj, E., Punamäki, R.-L., et al. (2009). Health in the occupied Palestinian territory 4 health as human security in the occupied Palestinian territory. *Lancet, 373*(9669), 1133–1143. doi:10.1016/s0140-6736(09)60110-0.

Bergman, L. R., von Eye, A., & Magnusson, D. (2006). Person-oriented research strategies in developmental psychopathology. In D. Cicchetti & D. J. Cohen (Eds.), *Developmental psychopathology* (2nd ed., pp. 850–888). Hoboken, NJ: Wiley.

Betancourt, T. S., Agnew-Blais, J., Gilman, S. E., Williams, D. R., & Ellis, B. H. (2010a). Past horrors, present struggles: The role of stigma in the association between war experiences and psychosocial adjustment among former child soldiers in Sierra Leone. *Social Science and Medicine, 70*(1), 17–26. doi:10.1016/j.socscimed.2009.09.038.

Betancourt, T. S., Borisova, I. I., Williams, T. P., Brennan, R. T., Whitfield, T. H., de la Soudiere, M., et al. (2010b). Sierra Leone's former child soldiers: A follow-up study of psychosocial adjustment and community reintegration. *Child Development, 81*(4), 1077–1095. doi:10.1111/j.1467-8624.2010.01455.x.

Betancourt, T. S., Brennan, R. T., Rubin-Smith, J., Fitzmaurice, G. M., & Gilman, S. E. (2010c). Sierra Leone's former child soldiers: A longitudinal study of risk, protective factors, and mental health. *Journal of the American Academy of Child and Adolescent Psychiatry, 49*(6), 606–615. doi:10.1016/j.jaac.2010.03.008.

Betancourt, T. S., McBain, R., Newnham, E. A., & Brennan, R. T. (2013). Trajectories of internalizing problems in war-affected Sierra Leonean youth: Examining conflict and post conflict factors. *Child Development, 84*(2), 455–470. doi:10.1111/j.1467-8624.2012.01861.x.

Betancourt, T. S., McBain, R., Newnham, E. A., & Brennan, R. T. (2014). Context matters: Community characteristics and mental health among war-affected youth in Sierra Leone. *Journal of Child Psychology and Psychiatry, 55*(3), 217–226. doi:10.1111/jccp.12131.

Betancourt, T. E., McBain, R. K., Newnham, E. A., & Brennan, R. T. (2015). The intergenerational impact of war: Longitudinal relationships between caregiver and child mental health in postconflict Sierra Leone. *Journal of Child Psychology and Psychiatry.* Advance online publication. doi:10.1111/jcpp.12389.

Betancourt, T. S., Newnham, E. A., McBain, R., & Brennan, R. T. (2013). Post-traumatic stress symptoms among former child soldiers in Sierra Leone: Follow-up study. *British Journal of Psychiatry, 203*(1), 196–202. doi:10.1192/bjp.bp.112.113514.

Bowlby, J. (1969). Attachment and loss. In *Loss* (Vol. 1). New York: Basic Books.

Bowlby, J. (1973). Attachment and loss. In *Separation* (Vol. 2). New York: Basic Books.

Boxer, P., Huesmann, L. R., Dubow, E. F., Landau, S. F., Gvirsman, S. D., Shikaki, K., et al. (2013). Exposure to violence across the social ecosystem and the development of aggression: A test of ecological theory in the Israeli-Palestinian conflict. *Child Development, 84*(1), 163–177. doi:10.1111/j.1467-8624.2012.01848.x.

Cole, D. A., & Maxwell, S. E. (2003). Testing mediational models with longitudinal data: Questions and tips in the use of structural equation modeling. *Journal of Abnormal Psychology, 112*(4), 558.

Cummings, E. M., Davies, P. T., & Campbell, S. B. (2000). *Developmental psychopathology and family process: Theory, research, and clinical implications*. New York: Guilford Press.

Cummings, E. M., Goeke-Morey, M. C., Merrilees, C. E., Taylor, L. K., & Shirlow, P. (2014). A social-ecological, process-oriented perspective on political violence and child development. *Child Development Perspectives, 8*(2), 82–89. doi:10.1111/cdep.12067.

Cummings, E. M., Merrilees, C. E., Schermerhorn, A. C., Goeke-Morey, M. C., Shirlow, P., & Cairns, E. (2011). Longitudinal pathways between political violence and child adjustment: The role of emotional security about the community in Northern Ireland. *Journal of Abnormal Child Psychology, 39*, 213–224. doi:10.1007/s10802-010-9457-3.

Cummings, E. M., Merrilees, C. E., Schermerhorn, A. C., Goeke-Morey, M. C., Shirlow, P., & Cairns, E. (2012). Political violence and child adjustment: Longitudinal tests of sectarian antisocial behavior, family conflict and insecurity as explanatory pathways. *Child Development, 83*(2), 461–468. doi:10.1111/j.1467-8624.2011.01720.x.

Cummings, E. M., Merrilees, C. E., Taylor, L. K., Goeke-Morey, M. C., & Shirlow, P. (in press). Emotional insecurity about the community: A dynamic, within-person mediator of child adjustment in contexts of political violence. *Development and Psychopathology*.

Cummings, E. M., Merrilees, C. E., Taylor, L. K., Shirlow, P., Goeke-Morey, M. C., & Cairns, E. (2013a). Longitudinal relations between sectarian and nonsectarian community violence and child adjustment in Northern Ireland. *Development and Psychopathology, 25*(3), 615–627. doi:10.1017/S0954579413000059.

Cummings, E. M., Taylor, L. K., Merrilees, C. E., Goeke-Morey, M. C., & Shirlow, P. (2016). Emotional insecurity in the family and community and youth delinquency in Northern Ireland: A person-oriented analysis across five waves. *Journal of Child Psychology and Psychiatry, 57*(1), 47–54.

Cummings, E. M., Taylor, L. K., Merrilees, C. E., Goeke-Morey, M. C., Shirlow, P., & Cairns, E. (2013b). Relations between political violence and child adjustment: A four-wave test of the role of emotional insecurity about community. *Developmental Psychology, 49*(12), 2212–2224. doi:10.1037/a0032309.

Cummings, E. M., & Valentino, K. V. (2015). Development psychopathology. In W. F. Overton & P. C. M. Molenaar (Eds.), *Theory and Method. Volume 1 of the Handbook of child psychology and developmental science*. (7th ed.) (pp. 566–606). Editor-in-Chief: Richard M. Lerner. NJ, Wiley: Hoboken.

Davies, P. T., & Cummings, E. M. (1994). Marital conflict and child adjustment—An emotional security hypothesis. *Psychological Bulletin, 116*(3), 387–411. doi:10.1037/0033-2909.116.3.387.

Dubow, E. F., Boxer, P., Huesmann, L. R., Shikaki, K., Landau, S., Gvirsman, S. D., et al. (2010). Exposure to conflict and violence across contexts: Relations to adjustment across Palestinian children. *Journal of Clinical Child and Adolescent Psychology, 39*(1), 103–116. doi:10.1080/15374410903401153.

Dubow, E. F., Huesmann, L. R., Boxer, P., Landau, S., Dvir, S., Shikaki, K., et al. (2012). Exposure to political conflict and violence and posttraumatic stress in Middle East youth: Protective factors. *Journal of Clinical Child and Adolescent Psychology, 41*(4), 402–416. doi:10.1080/15374416.2012.684274.

Goeke-Morey, M. C., Taylor, L. K., Merrilees, C. E., Shirlow, P., & Cummings, E. M. (2014). Adolescents' relationship with God and internalizing adjustment over time: The moderating role of maternal religious coping. *Journal of Family Psychology, 28*(6), 749–758. doi:10.1037/a0037170.

Hall, B. J., Tol, W. A., Jordans, M. J., Bass, J., & de Jong, J. T. (2014). Understanding resilience in armed conflict: Social resources and mental health of children in Burundi. *Social Science and Medicine, 114,* 121–128. doi:10.1016/j.socscimed.2014.05.042.

Haroz, E. E., Murray, L. K., Bolton, P., Betancourt, T., & Bass, J. K. (2013). Adolescent resilience in northern Uganda: The role of social support and prosocial behavior in reducing mental health problems. *Journal of Research on Adolescence, 23*(1), 138–148. doi:10.1111/j.1532-7795.2012.00802.x.

Hobfoll, S. E., Hall, B. J., Canetti-Nisim, D., Galea, S., Johnson, R. J., & Palmieri, P. A. (2007). Refining our understanding of traumatic growth in the face of terrorism: Moving from meaning cognitions to doing what is meaningful. *Applied Psychology: An International Review, 56*(3), 345–366. doi:10.1111/j.1464-0597.2007.00292.x.

Kuterovac-Jagodić, G. (2003). Posttraumatic stress symptoms in Croatian children exposed to war: A prospective study. *Journal of Clinical Psychology, 59*(1), 9–25. doi:10.1002/jclp.10114.

Maxwell, S. E., & Cole, D. A. (2007). Bias in cross-sectional analyses of longitudinal mediation. *Psychological methods, 12*(1), 23.

McAloney, K., McCrystal, P., Percy, A., & McCartan, C. (2009). Damaged youth: Prevalence of community violence exposure and implications for adolescent wellbeing in post-conflict Northern Ireland. *Journal of Community Psychology, 37*(5), 635–648. doi:10.1002/jcop.20322.

Merrilees, C. E., Cairns, E., Taylor, L. K., Goeke-Morey, M. C., Shirlow, P., & Cummings, E. M. (2013). Social identity and youth aggressive and delinquent behaviors in a context of political violence. *Political Psychology, 34*(5), 695–711. doi:10.1111/pops.12030.

Merrilees, C. E., Taylor, L. K., Goeke-Morey, M. C., Shirlow, P., & Cummings, E. M. (2014a). Youth in contexts of political violence: A developmental approach to the study of youth identity and emotional security in their communities. *Peace and Conflict: Journal of Peace Psychology, 20*(1), 26–39. doi:10.1080/10781910903088932.

Merrilees, C. E., Taylor, L. K., Goeke-Morey, M. C., Shirlow, P., Cummings, E. M., & Cairns, E. (2014b). The protective role of group identity: Sectarian antisocial behavior and adolescent emotion problems. *Child Development, 85*(1), 412–420. doi:10.1111/cdev.12125.

Palosaari, E., Punamäki, R.-L., Diab, M., & Qouta, S. (2013). Posttraumatic cognitions and posttraumatic stress symptoms among war-affected children: A cross-lagged analysis. *Journal of Abnormal Psychology, 122*(3), 656–661. doi:10.1037/a0033875.

Panter-Brick, C., Goodman, A., Tol, W., & Eggerman, M. (2011). Mental health and childhood adversities: A longitudinal study in Kabul, Afghanistan. *Journal of the American Academy of Child and Adolescent Psychiatry, 50*(4), 349–363. doi:10.1016/j.jaac.2010.12.001.

Punamäki, R.-L., Palosaari, E., Diab, M., Peltonen, K., & Qouta, S. R. (2015). Trajectories of posttraumatic stress symptoms (PTSS) after major war among Palestinian children: Trauma, family, and child-related predictors. *Journal of Affective Disorders, 172,* 133–140. doi:10.1016/j.jad.2014.09.021.

Sterba, S. K., & Bauer, D. J. (2010). Matching method with theory in person-oriented developmental psychopathology research. *Development and Psychopathology, 22*(2), 239–254. doi:10.1017/S0954579410000015.

Taylor, L. K., Merrilees, C. E., Goeke-Morey, M. C., Shirlow, P., & Cummings, E. M. (2014). Trajectories of adolescent aggression and family cohesion: The potential to perpetuate or ameliorate political conflict. *Journal of Clinical Child and Adolescent Psychology, 13*(1), 1–15. doi:10.1080/15374416.2014.945213.

Chapter 7
Tier 4: Prevention and Intervention Research

Keywords Translational research · Randomized clinical trials · Trauma-focused cognitive behavioral therapy · Teacher-delivered programs · Internalizing problems · Social support · Psychosocial interventions

Thus far this review has focused on basic research examining the impact of political violence and armed conflict on youth at the Tiers 1-3 levels. This section focuses on Tier 4, which is constituted by translational research (Cicchetti & Toth, 2006), that is, when basic research discoveries are applied to the development of more effective treatment and prevention models (Gunnar & Cicchetti, 2009; Insel, 2005; National Advisory Mental Health Council, 2000; Rubio et al., 2010; Zerhouni, 2003). As with other tiers of the pyramid, our goal is not to provide an exhaustive review, but rather to richly reflect the "state of the art" in prevention and intervention studies (see Table 7.1). This section begins with overall limitations and best practices for translational research in this field, presents our selection criteria for the studies reported in Table 7.1, and then reviews a number of important studies based on the levels of the social ecology.

Consistent with the urgency of the problems faced by youth, numerous efforts have been made to develop programs to foster well-being and mental health in contexts of political violence and armed conflict (e.g., Betancourt et al., 2013; Jordans, Tol, Komproe, & de Jong, 2009; Peltonen & Punamäki, 2010). However, in many cases, these programs have not been evaluated or met rigorous criteria of presentation of scientific evidence on program efficacy for psychosocial intervention or prevention programs. For example, many program evaluations have not utilized either random assignment procedures or control groups, nor evaluated the fidelity of program implementation or the sustainability of program effects. These limitations are challenging, but not insurmountable.

There are a number of best practices for rigorous translational research that are informed by a developmental psychopathology perspective. The first is the use of randomized clinical trials (RCTs). RCTs are considered the "gold standard" for evaluating the efficacy of prevention and intervention programs. The consensus among reviewers of this literature is that RCT evaluations of programs for youth

E.M. Cummings et al., *Political Violence, Armed Conflict, and Youth Adjustment*, DOI 10.1007/978-3-319-51583-0_7 affected by political violence and armed conflict are relatively few and far between (e.g., Betancourt et al., 2013; Jordans et al., 2009). A *randomly* assigned control group addresses the possibility that in universal programs, there may be an average zero-order change (e.g., net no change in outcomes), especially for trauma-related symptoms, which might be expected to improve over time for some youth. However, even in studies where an RCT design is employed, many lack a "no treatment" control group, which leaves open the possibility that identified improvements are due to placebo effects (e.g., the attention provided to participants in the treatment groups compared to control groups). Moreover, although waitlist control groups are appropriate to address concerns about participants not receiving treatment, reliance on waitlist controls inevitably limits the potential period for follow-up assessments, so that questions remain about whether treatment benefits are long-lasting.

The second best practice for translational research is that the study intervention components are designed from well-articulated theory, as well as basic research findings regarding mediating and moderating mechanisms (Borkowski, Smith, & Akai, 2007; Nation et al., 2003). The third best practice is that intervention outcomes should test both short- and long-term efficacy. Finally, especially pertinent to the study of youth in contexts of armed conflict, the fourth best practice is the identification of intervention components at multiple levels of the social ecology (Cicchetti & Toth, 2006; Gunner & Cicchetti, 2009).

For this review, the majority of the studies on intervention programs that we uncovered were identified during our previously described literature searches. Supplemental searches were also conducted on Web of Science and PsycINFO in autumn 2014, spring 2015, and summer 2015. These searches incorporated the above search terms, in conjunction with specific prevention and intervention-oriented search terms (e.g., "prevention"; "intervention"; "evaluation"; "program"; "randomized controlled trial"). Results were cross-checked with the reference lists of key and highly cited literature reviews and meta-analyses in this area. Forwards and backwards searches were also conducted on key and highly cited articles.

As with Tables 4.1, 5.1, 6.1, and 7.1 presents a sample of 20 prevention and intervention studies representing diverse geographic contexts and political conflicts, a range of independent and dependent variables, diverse youth populations, and multiple research groups. Moreover, the selected studies often included relatively large sample sizes, stronger sampling procedures, RCT designs, appropriate statistical analyses, and other evidence of methodological rigor or complexity. The criteria for an intervention to be classified as "translational research" are that the paper *explicitly* presented (a) clear evidence that the program was grounded in longitudinal, process-oriented research (Tiers 1–3) (denoted by "*"), or (b) clear evidence that the study was guided by a theoretical model (denoted by "+"). In addition to these distinctions, Table 7.1 includes information about the content and goals of the intervention to contextualize the results; sample sizes; whether comparisons are relative to baseline scores or control conditions; whether interventions occurred during periods of ongoing or post-accord conflict; measures employed; and major findings.

Table 7.1 Prevention and Intervention Studies

Region and conflict	Reference	Intervention	Sample and treatment groups	Assessment timing	Measures	Major findings
Africa						
Burundi; ongoing political instability and ethnic violence	Tol et al. (2014)*+	• 15 sessions of a manualized, school-based group intervention • Intervention incorporated trauma-processing activities, cooperative play, and creative expressive elements	• 329 youth (M age = 12.29 years) who had been exposed to at least one traumatic event and exhibited significant mental health symptoms • Cluster randomization to the intervention (n = 153) or waitlist control condition (n = 176)	• Three assessments: pre-intervention, 1 week; post-intervention; and 3 months post-intervention • Data collection occurred during a period of ongoing political instability and ethnic violence	• Exposure to traumatic events • PTSD • Hope • Coping repertoire • Coping satisfaction • Social support • Social capital	• No significant main effects of intervention were detected for PTSD, depressive, or anxiety symptoms (in relation to the control group) • In the intervention condition, participants living in larger households exhibited greater decreases on depressive symptoms and functional impairment across time-points • In the intervention group, participants living with both parents exhibited greater decreases on PTSD and depressive symptoms across time-points • Hope trajectories differed by study condition in interaction with age, traumatic exposure, and displacement status
Democratic Republic of the Congo; ongoing conflict	McMullen, O'Callaghan, Shannon, Black, and Eakin (2013)	• 15 sessions of manualized group trauma-focused cognitive behavioral therapy • Intervention-incorporated elements of cognitive and behavioral therapy	• 50 boys (M age at baseline = 15.8 years), including former child soldiers (n = 39) and other war-affected boys (n = 11) • Random assignment to the intervention (n = 25) or waitlist control group (n = 25)	• Three assessments at baseline, post-intervention, and 3-month follow-up • Data collection occurred during a period of ongoing conflict	• Exposure to traumatic war events • PTSD • Psychosocial distress, including depression/anxiety-like symptoms, conduct problems, and prosocial behavior	• Intervention participants exhibited reductions in PTSD symptoms, reductions in depression/anxiety-like symptoms, reductions in conduct problems, and increases in prosocial behavior at T2 compared to control group participants • Intervention effect sizes were greater for former child soldiers than other war-affected youth • Intervention-related gains were maintained at T3
Democratic Republic of the Congo; ongoing conflict	O'Callaghan et al. (2014)*	• Eight sessions of a manualized, thrice-weekly, group psychosocial intervention • Youth participated with one caregiver • Intervention-incorporated youth life skills leadership training; narrative films on stigma, discrimination, and reintegration in the family and community; and relaxation training drawn from trauma-focused cognitive behavioral therapy	• 159 youth (M age at baseline = 13.42 years) living in villages affected by high levels of violence • Random assignment of matched pair members into intervention (n = 79) or control groups (n = 80)	• Three assessments at pre-intervention, 4 weeks post-intervention, and 3 months post-intervention • Data collection occurred during a period of ongoing conflict	• Experiences with the Lord's Resistance Army (youth report) • PTSD (youth report) • Internalizing symptoms (youth report) • Conduct problems (youth and caregiver report) • Prosocial behavior (youth report)	• At T2, intervention group participants reported significantly fewer PTSD symptoms than control group members • At T3, members of both groups exhibited reductions in internalizing symptoms and conduct problems, and increases in prosocial behavior

(continued)

Table 7.1 (continued)

Region and conflict	Reference	Intervention	Sample and treatment groups	Assessment timing	Measures	Major findings
Democratic Republic of the Congo; ongoing conflict	O'Callaghan, McMullen, Shannon, and Rafferty (2015)	• Comparison of two interventions: trauma-focused cognitive behavioral therapy and the psychosocial Child Friendly Spaces program (both nine thrice-weekly sessions) • Trauma-focused cognitive behavioral therapy incorporated elements of cognitive and behavioral therapy to promote trauma processing and healing • Child Friendly Spaces incorporated creative, expressive, and discursive activities to teach participants about how to avoid common dangers	• 72 war-affected youth (M age = 14.79 years) • Randomization to the trauma-focused cognitive behavioral therapy group (n = 26), Child Friendly Spaces group (n = 24), or waitlist control group (n = 22)	• Three assessments at pre-intervention, post-intervention, and 6 months post-intervention • assessment timing?	• Adverse life events • PTSD • Internalizing symptoms • Conduct problems • Prosocial behavior	• Members of both intervention groups exhibited greater reductions in PTSD symptoms, internalizing and conduct problems between T1 and T3 than control group members • Participants of the Child Friendly Spaces intervention exhibited significant reductions in prosocial behavior at T3 compared to participants who received trauma-focused cognitive behavioral therapy
Sierra Leone; Sierra Leone Civil War	Gupta and Zimmer (2008)	• Four weeks of the teacher-delivered Rapid-Ed intervention, aimed at addressing displaced youths' educational needs and psychological distress • Intervention-incorporated basic literacy and numeracy education, structured trauma healing activities, and recreational activities	• 315 randomly selected displaced youth (M age = 10.7 years) • No control group	• Two assessments, pre-intervention and 4- to 6-week post-intervention • Data collection occurred several months after a rebel invasion in Sierra Leone	• Exposure to war violence • Impact of events and PTSD symptoms • Subjective feelings about the intervention's trauma healing activities	• Participants exhibited significant reductions in intrusion and arousal symptoms between T1 and T2 • Participants exhibited increases in optimism about the future and slight increases in avoidance reactions between T1 and T2
Sierra Leone; Sierra Leone Civil War	Newnham et al. (2015)[a]	• Ten weekly sessions of the manualized, group-based Youth Readiness Intervention • Intervention incorporated and training in relaxation, communication, cognitive restructuring, behavioral activation, goal setting, and problem solving	• 32 war-affected youth (ages 15–24 years) with ongoing psychological and behavioral problems • No control group	• Two assessments, pre- and post-intervention • Intervention was implemented after the war had ended	• Psychological symptoms • Functional adaptation • Emotion regulation • Intervention fidelity	• Participants exhibited reductions in internalizing symptoms, externalizing symptoms, and functional impairment between T1 and T2 • Participants exhibited improvements in emotion regulation, adaptive behavior, and quality of life between T1 and T2
Asia						
Indonesia; ongoing communal violence	Tol et al. (2008)	• 15 sessions of a manualized, school-based group intervention • Intervention incorporated trauma-processing activities, cooperative play, and creative expressive elements	• 495 youth (M age = 9.9 years) • 81.4% of participants were included • Cluster randomization to the intervention (n = 182) or waitlist control conditions (n = 221)	• Three assessments, 1 week pre-intervention, 1 week post-intervention, and 6 months post-intervention • Data collection occurred during a period of ongoing conflict	• Exposure to violent events (youth report) • PTSD (youth report) • Depression (youth report) • Anxiety (youth report) • Aggression (parent report) • Hope (youth report)	• After correcting for clustering, treatment recipients exhibited greater maintenance of hope and reductions in PTSD symptoms across time-points than control group members • Treatment recipients did not exhibit significant reductions in traumatic stress-related symptoms, depressive symptoms, anxiety symptoms, or functional impairment across time-points compared to control group members

(continued)

Table 7.1 (continued)

Region and conflict	Reference	Intervention	Sample and treatment groups	Assessment timing	Measures	Major findings
Indonesia; ongoing communal violence	Tol et al. (2010)	• 15 sessions of a manualized, school-based group intervention • Intervention incorporated trauma-processing activities, cooperative play, and creative expressive elements	• 403 youth (M age = 9.9 years) who had been exposed to at least one political violence event and were exhibiting mental health symptoms • Cluster randomization to the treatment (n = 182) or waitlist control condition (n = 221)	• Three assessments: pre-intervention, 1 week post-intervention, and 6 months post-intervention • Data collection occurred during a period of ongoing conflict	• Exposure to traumatic events (youth report) • PTSD (youth report) • Hope (youth report) • Coping skills (youth report) • Coping satisfaction (youth report) • Social support (youth report) • Family connectedness (parent report) • Functional impairment (youth and parent report)	• Treatment recipients exhibited increased positive coping, increased play social support, greater maintenance of hope, and greater maintenance of peer social support across time-points compared to control group members • Play social support mediated the effects of treatment on PTSD, such that increases in play social support were related to smaller reductions in symptoms in the treatment group • Gender, household size, and social support moderated some outcomes in the treatment group
Israel; ongoing conflict	Berger, Pat-Horenczyk, and Gelkopf (2007)	• Eight sessions of Overshadowing the Threat of Terrorism, a teacher-led intervention • Intervention incorporated psychoeducation, meditative practice, bio-energy exercises, art therapy, and narrative techniques	• 142 youth (Grades 2–6) • Cluster randomization to the intervention or waitlist control conditions • 33–51% of the pupils in each classroom participated in the assessment (intervention n = 70; waitlist control n = 72)	• Two assessments, pre-intervention and 2 months post-intervention • Data collection occurred during a period of ongoing conflict, in the aftermath of recent terror attacks	• Objective exposure to terrorism • Subjective exposure to terrorism • PTSD • Functional impairment • Somatic problems • Generalized anxiety • Separation anxiety	• Intervention participants exhibited greater reductions in functional impairment, somatic problems, depressive symptoms and PTSD severity between T1 and T2 than control group members
Israel; ongoing conflict	Gelkopf and Berger (2009)	• Twelve weekly sessions of ERASE-Stress, a manualized teacher-delivered intervention • Intervention-incorporated psychoeducation, skill training, meditative practices, and narrative techniques	• 114 war-affected youth (M age at baseline = 13.05 years) • Random assignment to the intervention (n = 58) or waitlist control group (n = 49)	• Two assessments, pre-intervention and 3 months post-intervention • Data collection occurred during a period of ongoing conflict	• Objective exposure to terror attacks • Subjective exposure/emotional reactions to terror attacks • PTSD • Functional impairment • Somatic problems • Depression • Program reliability and consistency	• Intervention participants exhibited greater reductions in functional impairment, somatic problems, depressive symptoms and PTSD severity between T1 and T2 than control group members
Israel; Operation Cast Lead and ongoing conflict	Slone, Shoshani, and Lobel (2013)*	• Six-week, manualized, teacher-delivered primary prevention program aimed at promoting self-efficacy and support mobilization • Program-incorporated group activities, discussions, and multimedia presentations	• 179 youth (M age = 16.3 years) exposed to high or low levels of political life events • School classes were randomly assigned to intervention (n = 94) or control conditions (n = 85)	• Two assessments: pre- and post-intervention • Intervention began 1 week after ceasefire declaration	• Exposure to political life events • Psychological symptoms • Psychological difficulties • Prosocial behavior • Social support	• Intervention participants exhibited increased ability to mobilize social support, increased self-efficacy, and decreased mental health symptoms between T1 and T2 compared to control group members

(continued)

Table 7.1 (continued)

Region and conflict	Reference	Intervention	Sample and treatment groups	Assessment timing	Measures	Major findings
					• Self-efficacy	• Intervention effects were evident among participants from both the high- and low-PLE groups
Israel; Second Lebanon War	Wolmer, Hamiel, Barchas, Slone, and Laor (2011)	• Fifteen weekly, manualized, teacher-delivered sessions focused on enhancing coping and socio-emotional skills and alleviating trauma • Intervention content was presented via letters from an imaginary character who shares his experiences, emotions, and coping strategies	• 983 intervention group participants (ages 8–12 years) • 1,152 youth comprised a matched, non-randomized waitlist control group, completing their baseline assessments at T3	• Three assessments at pre-intervention (5 months post-war), post-intervention (9 months post-war), and post-intervention (12 months post-war)	• Stressful life events before the war (parent report) • Fear, stress, and mood (youth report) • Classroom atmosphere (teacher report) • Concerns about children's school performance, social and family functioning, stress/anxiety, health, and mood (parent report)	• Intervention participants exhibited significant decreases in PTSD, stress, and mood symptoms between T1 and T2 compared to control group members • Intervention participants exhibited significantly fewer PTSD symptoms at T3 than control group members
Lebanon; Operation Grapes of Wrath	Karam et al. (2008)	• Twelve consecutive days of a manualized teacher-delivered intervention • Intervention incorporated cognitive behavioral and stress inoculation training	• 2,500 youth received the intervention, which was mandated at their schools; 116 were randomly selected for the intervention evaluation (M age at baseline = 11.7 and 11.8 years for treatment and control participants, respectively) • Youth from different schools where the intervention was not implemented served as the control group (n = 93) • Intervention and control groups were not matched	• Two assessments: 1 month post-war (pre-intervention), and 1 year post-war • Intervention was implemented post-war	• Exposure to war events (parent report) • Depression • Separation anxiety • PTSD • Psychosocial stressors	• There were no significant intervention effects on rates of depression, separation anxiety disorder, or PTSD • Pre-war separation anxiety disorder and PTSD, family violence, financial problems, and exposure to war events predicted psychological disorders at T2
Nepal; Nepalese Civil War	Jordans et al. (2010)	• Fifteen sessions of the 5-week classroom-based intervention • Intervention-incorporated elements of creative expressive and experiential therapy, cooperative play and cognitive behavioral therapy	• 325 youth (M age at baseline = 12.7 years) • Cluster randomization to the intervention (n = 164) or waitlist control group (n = 161)	• Two assessments at pre-intervention and post-intervention • T1 data collection occurred approximately 1 to 2 months post-war • T2 data collection occurred approximately 4 months post-war	• Psychological distress • PTSD • Depression • Sub-clinical psychological problems • Anxiety • Functional impairment • Hope • Prosocial behavior • Aggression	• Boys in the intervention group exhibited greater reductions in psychological problems and aggression between T1 and T2 compared to control group members • Girls in the intervention group exhibited greater increases in prosocial behavior between T1 and T2 compared to control group members • Older children in the intervention group exhibited greater increases in hope between T1 and T2 compared to control group members

(continued)

Table 7.1 (continued)

Region and conflict	Reference	Intervention	Sample and treatment groups	Assessment timing	Measures	Major findings
Palestine; Gaza War and ongoing conflict	Diab, Peltonen, Qouta, Palosaari, and Punamäki (2015)	• Sixteen extracurricular sessions of the manualized teaching recovery techniques intervention • Intervention incorporated trauma-related psychoeducation, cognitive behavioral therapy strategies, coping skills training, and creative expressive elements	• 482 youth (M age at baseline = 11.29 years) • Cluster randomization to the intervention (n = 242) or waitlist control conditions (n = 240)	• Three assessments at pre-intervention, 2 months post-intervention, and 6 months post-intervention • Intervention began three-and-a-half months post-war	• Exposure to traumatic events • Psychosocial well-being • Prosocial behavior • Maternal attachment • Family atmosphere	• Resilience was conceptualized as the presence of positive indicators of mental health, despite exposure to traumatic events • Intervention participants did not exhibit significant increases in resilience between time-points compared to the control group members • Neither maternal attachment nor family atmosphere moderated intervention effects
Palestine; ongoing conflict	Peltonen, Qouta, El Sarraj, and Punamäki (2010)	• Academic year-long implementation of the School Mediation Intervention, led by teachers and older students • Intervention incorporated training in self-regulation, problem solving, conflict resolution, and dialogue skills	• 225 youth (M age at baseline = 11.37 years) • Classrooms were randomly selected from schools where the intervention was being implemented (n youth = 141) and was not (n youth = 84)	• Two assessments: pre-intervention and immediately post-intervention • Data collection and the intervention were conducted during a period of ongoing conflict	• Military trauma • PTSD • Depression • Psychological distress • Friendship quality • Prosocial behavior • Aggression	• Intervention participants did not exhibit significant reductions in symptoms, increases in friendship quality, prosocial behavior, or non-aggressive behavior between T1 and T2 compared to control group members • Intervention participants exhibited less deterioration of friendships and prosocial behavior between T1 and T2 compared to control group members
Palestine; Gaza War and ongoing conflict	Qouta, Palosaari, Diab, and Punamäki (2012)	• Sixteen twice-weekly extracurricular sessions of the teaching recovery techniques intervention • Intervention incorporated trauma-related psychoeducation, cognitive behavioral therapy strategies, coping skills training, and creative-expression elements	• 482 youth (M age at baseline = 11.29 years) • Cluster randomization to the intervention (n = 242) or waitlist control conditions (n = 240)	• Three assessments at pre-intervention, post-intervention, and 6 months post-intervention • Intervention began several months post-war	• Peri-traumatic dissociation • PTSD • Depression • Psychological distress	• The proportion of clinical PTSD symptoms was significantly reduced among boys in the intervention group between T1 and T2, compared to the control group • Girls in the intervention group with low levels of peri-traumatic dissociation exhibited reductions in PTSD symptoms and the proportion of clinically significant PTSD symptoms between T1 and T2 compared to control group members
Sri Lanka; Sri Lankan Civil War	Tol et al. (2012)	• 15 sessions of a manualized, school-based group intervention • Intervention incorporated trauma-processing activities, cooperative play, and creative expressive elements	• 399 youth (M age = 11.03 years) • Cluster randomization to the intervention (n = 199) or waitlist control condition (n = 200)	• Three assessments: pre-intervention, 1 week post-intervention, and 3 months post-intervention • Data collection occurred during a period of ongoing conflict	• Exposure to violence • Daily stressors • PTSD • Depression • Anxiety • Psychological difficulties • Prosocial behavior • Supernatural complaints • War-related conduct problems	• No significant intervention effects were detected for PTSD, depressive, or anxiety symptoms • Intervention participants, especially younger ones, exhibited greater reductions in conduct problems across time-points than control group members • Some subgroup effects were detected for intervention benefits over time by gender, age, and levels of ongoing war-related stressors

(continued)

Table 7.1 (continued)

Region and conflict	Reference	Intervention	Sample and treatment groups	Assessment timing	Measures	Major findings
					• Functional impairment • Coping repertoire and satisfaction	
Europe						
Bosnia and Herzegovina; Bosnian War	Layne et al. (2008)	• Two tiers of a school- and community-based mental health program • First tier was a classroom-based psychoeducation and skills intervention (active-treatment comparison condition) • Second tier was a 17–20 weekly group sessions of trauma- and grief-focused treatment, paired with the classroom intervention (treatment condition)	• 127 youth who were severely affected by the war • Participants were randomly assigned to either the treatment ($n = 66$) or comparison group ($n = 61$)	• Assessments at pre-treatment, post-treatment, and 4 months post-treatment • Assessments were conducted several years post-war	• Exposure to trauma and severe adversity before, during, and after the war • PTSD • Depression • Maladaptive grief reactions	• Members of both groups exhibited reductions in PTSD and depression symptoms between T1 and T2, and T3 • Treatment recipients, but not control group members, exhibited significant reductions in maladaptive grief reactions between T1 and T2
Croatia; Croatian War of Independence	Woodside, Barbara, and Benner (1999)	• Four months of weekly, teacher-delivered sessions • Intervention-incorporated educational lessons on traumatic healing, non-violent conflict resolution, peaceful living, awareness of human rights and ethnic bias	• 251 youth (M age = 11.9 years) • Three classrooms received the intervention treatment ($n = 97$) • Three classrooms were in the same schools as the intervention group but did not receive the intervention, serving as a semi-control group • Three classrooms did not receive the intervention, serving as the control group	• Three assessments: pre-intervention, post-intervention, and one year post-intervention • Intervention was delivered approximately 2–6 months post-war	• Exposure to traumatic events • PTSD • Depression • Self-esteem • Self-concept • Conflict resolution practices • Social skills • Attitudes and beliefs toward conflict resolution • Psychosocial classroom climate • Social distance scale (measuring ethnic bias) • Ethnic attitudes • Academic grades	• Intervention participants exhibited greater reductions in PTSD symptoms between T1 and T2, and T2 and T3 than control group members • Intervention participants exhibited greater positive change in ethnic attitudes over time than control group members

*Clear indication in the journal article that the prevention or intervention program is grounded in longitudinal, process-oriented research. If unclear, * designation was not made
+Clear indication in the journal article that the study was guided by a theoretical model. If unclear, + designation was not made

We will now briefly review evidence for the significance of prevention and intervention programs targeting different levels of the social ecology.

Individual characteristics. Approaches targeting individual functioning hold promise for directly affecting youth functioning and adjustment. For example, McMullen et al. (2013) conducted an RCT with former child soldiers and other boys affected by war in the Democratic Republic of Congo. This is an example of a treatment program that was developed with American youth exposed to violence being extended to youth exposed to armed conflict in another country. Although it is ideal to have Tier 3 research to rely on for program development, in the absence of that, adapting evidence-based programs for US youth exposed to violence merit consideration, given the urgency of the problems faced by youth. In McMullen and colleagues' intervention, participants were randomly assigned to a treatment group, which received 15 group-based sessions of a manualized psychological treatment, trauma-focused cognitive behavioral therapy, or to a waitlist control group. Treatment group members exhibited significant reductions in mental health symptoms, as well as increases in prosocial behaviors, relative to control group members. These effects were maintained at a 3-month follow-up of the treatment group (see O'Callaghan, McMullen, Shannon, Rafferty, & Black, 2013, for the results of a similar trial with girls). This intervention showed promising results, including improvements on a broad range of outcomes, in the context of a rigorous research design that revealed sustained impact over time compared to a waitlist control group.

Rather than adapting an existing intervention from a Western model, other studies have aimed to provide more culturally grounded interventions. Newnham et al. (2015) conducted a feasibility study for a group mental health treatment, the Youth Readiness Intervention, for war-affected youth in Sierra Leone. Because this approach was explicitly informed by longitudinal and qualitative studies by the same research group in Sierra Leone, and by elements of cognitive behavioral therapy, it may be regarded as a Tier 4 study. The program adapted a cognitively based intervention to address the multiple challenges and mental health needs and challenges of war-affected youth. Based on Newnham and colleagues' initial feasibility study, the results appear promising for reducing internalizing and externalizing symptoms. Limitations of this study include the non-RCT design, small sample size, and lack of screening specifically for direct exposure to political violence.

Despite some limitations, both of these studies represent examples of interventions that incorporate many of the best practices in translational research to influence individual youth adjustment in settings of armed conflict.

Microsystem factors: Family. The family constitutes a microsystem context that is relatively proximal to youth functioning and which therefore may have high impact on youth adjustment (Cummings, Davies, & Campbell, 2000). The Tier 4 literature suggests that family functioning may be amenable to change even in contexts of intransient and ongoing political violence. In an example of a family-level intervention, Dybdahl (2001) evaluated the impact of an RCT psychosocial intervention program for mothers on their children. The weekly intervention was conducted over five months. Giving that the intervention took place 6 months following the end of the war in Bosnia and Herzegovina, the program was initially informed by trauma discussion groups for mothers that were conducted during the war and then developed based on the literature on the importance of mother–child interaction for children's coping with stress (e.g., information derived from the International Child Development Program). Comparing changes from pre-test to post-test changes in intervention and nonintervention control groups by means of t-tests, the results indicated significant effects on some indices of mothers' and children's mental health and psychosocial functioning.

In another example of a family-focused intervention, O'Callaghan et al. (2014) employed a group-based (matched-pair design) RCT approach in the Democratic Republic of the Congo. The intervention included community seminars to evaluate a psychosocial intervention with elements drawn from multiple sources (e.g., a youth life skills program developed in Tanzania, relaxation training scripts, a cinema program addressing themes of stigma and discrimination for former child soldiers). Although improvements within the intervention conditions were identified at post-test (e.g., reduced PTSD symptoms), a three-month follow-up (e.g., reduced internalizing symptoms) showed limited evidence of benefits relative to the control group. The overall impact of the study is also limited by the lack of clear evidence of translation of specific elements of basic research and corresponding testing of models for why or how the program was effective.

Reflecting the many practical and logistical challenges for constructing large-scale prevention and interventions studies, relatively few family-focused interventions have been tested. The relative dearth of robust interventions at this level of the social ecology leaves many questions remaining for future research. Notably, limitations of research focused only on the family include the limitations associated with testing only one level of the social ecology, and such interventions are relatively expensive and time-consuming to accomplish.

Microsystem factors: Schools. The most frequent context for interventions for youth affected by political violence is schools, with them majority focusing on internalizing symptoms. For example, Slone, Shoshani, and Lobel (2013) led a school-based, teacher-delivered program that was derived from psychiatric and psychological literatures on support mobilization and self-efficacy. In this intervention, social support and self-efficacy in coping with stress was linked with pre-test to post-test improvements in these processes, and both constructs reduced psychological distress compared to a waitlist control group. The importance of social support was also found in a school-based psychosocial intervention in Indonesia (Tol et al., 2010). In an innovative effort at testing mediators and moderators, results suggested that social support mediated reductions in PTSD symptoms and that various characteristics moderated treatment outcomes (e.g., child gender). These studies suggest that social support, which has the potential to cross levels of the social ecology, may be effectively targeted in some school-based interventions.

Among the notable examples of extensive school program development and evaluation, Gelkopf and Berger (2009) reported that Israeli students who participated in a 12-session classroom intervention (ERASE-Stress) exhibited significant reductions in mental health symptoms at a three-month follow-up relative to a waitlist control group. The program began with seven three-hour sessions of teacher training and included psycho-educational information, skills practice, and experiential exercises. The program also included classroom simulations in which the elements of the program were practiced and evaluated, and three two-hour sessions in which issues of application were raised and possible solutions were discussed. The youth component of ERASE-Stress administered by teachers involved twelve 90-min classroom sessions that included presentation of psychoeducational material, experience and closure exercises, and coverage of multiple topics (e.g., controlling your emotions, knowing your feelings). Parents also attended two psychoeducational sessions at the outset of the program. The same research group also reported significant reductions in PTSD symptoms among Israeli participants relative to a quasi-randomized, wait-list control condition in a 16-session version of ERASE-Stress (Berger, Gelkopf, & Heineberg, 2012). Groups were assigned by picking paper slips out of a bag and assigning two classrooms to the treatment condition for each classroom that was assigned to the control condition.

Several other studies have reported on interventions that effectively reduced youth mental health symptoms in contexts of political violence. For example, in Bosnia, Layne et al. (2008) implemented an RCT in which all participating youth received a classroom-based psychoeducational and skills intervention, and about half additionally received trauma and grief component therapy for war-exposed adolescents. Rates of PTSD and depressive symptoms decreased among the members of both the treatment and comparison groups; however, the percentage of participants who exhibited substantial reductions in symptoms was relatively higher in the treatment group. A notable point in this study was the use of an active control group. After the Second Lebanon War in Israel, Wolmer et al. (2011) reported on a 16-week school-based intervention program consisting of 45-min, teacher-delivered modules aimed at promoting resilience. They found that treatment group members exhibited lower PTSD symptoms than control group members three months after program completion. However, the control group was not randomized, and measures were brief questionnaires that reflected only a subset of the standard items for included scales. Overall, despite variability in the strength of the research designs, this set of studies suggest that school-based interventions may be effective at improving mental health among youth in settings of political violence.

Other studies, however, have found more nuanced and mixed results in terms of the efficacy of school-based interventions to affect youth mental health. In Gaza, posttraumatic stress symptoms (PTSS) were targeted using a 16-week, teacher-delivered psychosocial intervention, including trauma-related psychoeducation, cognitive behavioral therapy strategies, coping skills training, and creative expression elements (Qouta et al. 2012). The intervention group exhibited reductions in PTSS from T1 to T2; however, there was no significant difference in PTSS change compared to the control group. There was also evidence that these effects were moderated by gender and baseline PTSS. That is, the intervention was not effective in reducing symptoms for boys, and among girls, only those with low levels of baseline PTSS showed reductions over time. In another context of intense periodic ethnic violence, Tol et al. (2014) evaluated the effectiveness of a 15-session school-based program in Burundi, assessing functioning before and after (1-week and 3 months) the intervention. Although no main effects were found, longitudinal growth curve analyses revealed relatively complex effects of moderated mediation, suggesting that preventive benefits may be contingent upon individual (e.g., gender) and contextual (e.g., family functioning) factors. In another study of a school-based intervention in Indonesia, Tol et al. (2008) reported evidence for reduction in PTSD symptoms for girls exposed to political violence, as well as some evidence for beneficial effects for boys (e.g., retained hope). However, these results should be interpreted in light of the study's use of assessors that were not blinded to treatment status. These studies highlight the need for analyses to consider potential individual and contextual moderators to evaluate program efficacy across diverse samples.

A number of other studies have reported less- or non-significant effects of school-based programs on a range of youth outcomes. For example, Jordans et al. (2010) reported on a 15-session school-based psychosocial intervention that incorporated the elements of creative expression and experiential therapy, cooperative play, and cognitive therapy for conflict-exposed youth in Nepal. Notably, analyses used appropriate procedures to control for nesting within schools. Although there were no significant reductions in psychiatric symptoms, evidence emerged for moderate, short-term, gender-specific benefits on some dimensions of psychosocial functioning (e.g., increased positive coping, maintained peer support) for the intervention group, relative to a waitlist control group. However, similar approaches in a Palestinian sample exposed to war in Gaza did not yield positive effects for youth outcomes. Diab et al. (2015) found that their school-based intervention (see Qouta et al., 2012) did not significantly increase resiliency, which was conceptualized as the presence of positive indicators of mental health despite exposure to traumatic events. This study was one of the few studies reviewed that included family measures, and the results did not find support for maternal attachment or family atmosphere moderating the impact of the classroom-based intervention.

Finally, not all reviewed studies found significant results for mental health outcomes. Working in post-war south Lebanese villages, Karam et al. (2008) reported on a teacher-delivered intervention that incorporated cognitive behavioral and stress inoculation training, and which was rooted this research group's earlier work with youth exposed to community violence. The intervention occurred on 12 consecutive school days. Youth rates of major depression, separation anxiety, and PTSD decreased from 1 month (pre-intervention) to one year post-war; however, these effects were non-significant. Limitations included the lack of randomized treatment or control groups, the provision of only brief training for teachers, and the assessment of fidelity of implementation through therapy diaries that were written by teachers who administered the program.

Advantages of a school-based intervention approach are that it facilitates data collection with relatively large sample sizes and targets an important level of youths' social ecologies. However, despite the fact that treatment benefits were reported in many of the studies that were reviewed, findings were often inconsistent across studies and qualified by post hoc moderators. Another note of caution is also warranted: Some reviews of school-based interventions have found evidence for increased psychological problems among some participants (Persson & Rousseau, 2009; Tol, Song, & Jordans, 2013). Despite the promises of this type of intervention, school environments in middle- and low-income countries may be unstable, informal, or limited by scarce resources, and these precarious settings may affect the efficacy of interventions (Tol et al., 2012, 2014). Significant questions thus remain about the sufficiency of school-based interventions as a stand-alone approach.

Summary

This review highlights the rich variety of directions towards providing urgently needed prevention and intervention programs for youth exposed to political violence and armed conflict. This literature begins to provide multiple possible directions for improving the adjustment and well-being of youth exposed to these circumstances, including programs targeting different levels of the social ecology (e.g., individual characteristics, family, and schools). Selected from the strongest programs according to our criteria, Table 7.1 provides rich detail about extant programs in multiple regions of the world, including research designs, outlines of intervention contents, assessment timing, and major findings. Moreover, programs approaching or meeting criteria for translational research are identified.

However, even among these relatively extensive programs, which show important effects for youth development in contexts of political violence, few reflect truly translational programs as they do not *explicitly* (a) test a theoretical model and/or (b) state how they are grounded in longitudinal, process-oriented research (Tiers 1–3). This limitation is also evident in other programs not meeting our selection criteria for Table 7.1. For example, programs based on group interpersonal psychotherapy in Northern Uganda (Bolton et al., 2007), "emergency education" in Chechnya (Betancourt, 2005), a "writing intervention" in Gaza (Lange-Nielsen et al., 2012), a participatory project based on Child Led Indicators in Nepal (Karki, Kohrt, & Jordans, 2009), and a 10-session-mind-body groups skills program in Gaza (Staples, Atti, & Gordon, 2011). Nonetheless, Table 7.1 represents recent efforts to posit and test psychological models for program effectiveness, with further advances also being made in approaches to randomization, based on cluster randomized trials (Tol et al., 2010, 2012, 2014) and randomization by classrooms rather than schools (Slone et al., 2013).

A prevalent alternative approach is program development based on "consensus-based guidelines," which are broad principles of intervention services to address mental health and psychosocial support needs (e.g., IASC Guidelines on Mental Health and Social Support in Emergency Settings, 2007). For example, these manualized interventions may contain a multilayered package of services, including cognitive behavior techniques (psychoeducation, coping programs) and creative expressive elements (e.g., song and dance, structured movement). However, little rigorous evidence is available to support the efficacy of these programs and high heterogeneity of effects is evident across programs (Tol et al., 2014). In addition, given the wide-range of program contents, it is difficult to evaluate the efficacy of specific elements of this consensus. This ambiguity highlights the urgency of identifying mediators and moderators of outcomes in order to understand how, why, and when programs work (Ertl & Neuner, 2014; Tol et al., 2014).

References

Berger, R., Pat-Horenczyk, R., & Gelkopf, M. (2007). School-based intervention for prevention and treatment of elementary-students' terror-related distress in Israel: A quasi-randomized controlled trial. *Journal of Traumatic Stress, 20*(4), 541–551. doi:10.1022/jts.

Berger, R., Gelkopf, M., & Heineberg, Y. (2012). A teacher-delivered intervention for adolescents exposed to ongoing and intense traumatic war-related stress: A quasi-randomized controlled study. *Journal of Adolescent Health, 51*(5), 453–461. doi:10.1016/j.jadohealth.2012.02.011.

Betancourt, T. S. (2005). Stressors, supports and the social ecology of displacement: Psychsocial dimensions of an emergency education program for Chechen adolescents displaced in Ingushetia, Russia. *Culture, Medicine and Psychiatry, 29*(3), 309–340. doi:10.1007/s11013-005-9170-9.

Betancourt, T. S., Borisova, I., Williams, T. P., Meyers-Ohki, S. E., Rubin-Smith, J. E., Annan, J., & Kohrt, B. A. (2013). Research review: Psychosocial adjustment and mental health in former child soldiers—A systematic review of the literature and recommendations for future research. *Journal of Child Psychology and Psychiatry, 54*(1), 17–36. doi:10.1111/j.1469-7610.2012.02620.x.

Bolton, P., Bass, J., Betancourt, T., Speelman, L., Onyango, G., Clougherty, K. F., ... Verdeli, H. (2007). Interventions for depression symptoms among adolescent survivors of war and displacement in Northern Uganda: A randomized controlled trial. *Journal of the American Medical Association, 298*(5), 519–527. doi:10.1001/jama.298.5.519.

Borkowski, J. G., Smith, L. E., & Akai, C. E. (2007). Designing effective prevention programs: How good science makes good art. *Infants and Young Children, 20*, 229–241.

Cicchetti, D., & Toth, S. L. (2006). Building bridges and crossing them: Translational research in developmental psychopathology. *Development and Psychopathology, 18*(3), 619–622. doi:10.1017/S0954579406060317.

Cummings, E. M., Davies, P. T., & Campbell, S. B. (2000). *Developmental psychopathology and family process: Theory, research, and clinical implications*. New York: Guilford Press.

Diab, M., Peltonen, K., Qouta, S. R., Palosaari, E., & Punamäki, R.-J. (2015). Effectiveness of psychosocial intervention enhancing resilience among war-affected children and the moderating role of family factors. *Child Abuse and Neglect, 40*, 24–35. doi:10.1016/j.chiabu.2014.12.002.

Dybdhal, R. (2001). Children and mothers in war: An outcome study of a psychosocial intervention program. *Child Development, 72*(4), 1214–1230. doi:10.1111/1467-8624.00343.

Ertl, V., & Neuner, F. (2014). Are school-based mental health interventions for war-affected children effective and harmless? *BMC Medicine, 12*(84). Add more. doi:10.1186/1741-7015-12-84.

Gelkopf, M., & Berger, R. (2009). A school-based, teacher-mediated prevention program (ERASE-Stress) for reducing terror-related traumatic reactions in Israeli youth: A quasi-randomized controlled trial. *Journal of Child Psychology and Psychiatry, 50*(8), 962–971. doi:10.1111/j.1469-7610.2008.02021.x.

Gunnar, M. R., & Cicchetti, D. (2009). Meeting the challenge of translational research in child psychology. In M. R. Gunnar & D. Cicchetti (Eds.), *Meeting the challenge of translational research in child psychology: Minnesota symposia on child psychology* (Vol. 35, pp. 1–27). New York: Wiley.

Gupta, L., & Zimmer, C. (2008). Psychosocial intervention for war-affected children in Sierra Leone. *The British Journal of Psychiatry, 192*, 212–216. doi:10.1192/bjp.bp.107.038182.

Insel, T. R. (2005). Developmental psychobiology for public health: A bridge for translational research. *Developmental Psychobiology, 47*(3), 209–216. doi:10.1002/dev.20089.

Inter-Agency Standing Committee. (2007). IASC Guidelines on mental health and social support in emergency settings. Retrieved, from http://www.who.int/mental_health/emergencies/guidelines_iasc_mental_health_psychosocial_june_2007.pdf.

Jordans, M. J. D., Komproe, I. H., Tol, W. A., Kohrt, B. A., Luitel, N. P., Macy, R. D., & de Jong, J. T. V. M. (2010). Evaluation of a classroom-based psychosocial intervention in conflict-affected Nepal: A cluster randomized controlled trial. *Journal of Child Psychology and Psychiatry, 51*(7), 818–826. doi:10.1111/j.1469-7610.2010.02209.x.

Jordans, M. J. D., Tol, W. A., Komproe, I. H., & de Jong, J. V. T. M. (2009). Systematic review of evidence and treatment approaches: Psychosocial and mental health care for children in war. *Child and Adolescent Mental Health, 14*(1), 2–14. doi:10.1111/j.1475-3588.2008.00515.x.

Karam, E. G., Fayyad, J., Karam, A. N., Tabet, C. C., Melhem, N., Mneimneh, M., & Dimassi, H. (2008). Effectiveness and specificity of a classroom-based group intervention in children and adolescents exposed to war in Lebanon. *World Psychiatry, 7*(2), 103–109. doi:10.1002/j.2051-5545.2008.tb00170.x.

Karki, R., Kohrt, B. A., & Jordans, M. J. (2009). Child led indicators: Pilot testing a child participation tool for psychosocial support programmes for former child soldiers in Nepal. *Intervention: Journal of Mental Health and Psychosocial Support in Conflict Affected Areas, 7*(2), 92–109. doi:10.1097/WTF.0b013e3283302725.

Lange-Nielsen, I. I., Kolltveit, S., Thabet, A. A. M., Dyregrov, A., Pallesen, S., Johnsen, T. B., & Laberg, J. C. (2012). Short-term effects of a writing intervention among adolescents in Gaza. *Journal of Loss and Trauma, 17*(5), 403–422. doi:10.1080/15325024.2011.650128.

Layne, C. M., Saltzman, W. R., Poppleton, L., Burlingame, G. M., Pašalić, A., Duraković, E., ... Pynooos, R. S. (2008). Effectiveness of a school-based group psychotherapy program for war-exposed adolescents: A randomized controlled trial. *Journal of the American Academy of Child and Adolescent Psychiatry, 47*(9), 1048–1062. doi:10.1097/CHI.0b013e31817eecae.

McMullen, J., O'Callaghan, P., Shannon, C., Black, A., & Eakin, J. (2013). Group trauma-focused cognitive-behavioural therapy with former child soldiers and other war-affected boys in the DR Congo: A randomized controlled trial. *Journal of Child Psychology and Psychiatry, 54*(11), 1231–1241. doi:10.1111/jccp.12094.

Nation, M., Crusto, C., Wanderman, A., Kumofer, K. L., Sevbolt, D., & Morrissey, K. E., et al. (2003). What works in prevention?: Principles of effective prevention programs. *American Psychologist, 58*, 229–456.

National Advisory Mental Health Council. (2000). *Translating behavioral science into action: Report of the National Advisory Mental Health Council's behavioral science workgroup* (no. 00–4699). Bethesda, MD: National Institutes of Mental Health.

Newnham, E. A., McBain, R. K., Hann, K., Akinsulure-Smith, A. M., Weisz, J., Lilienthal, G. M., ... Betancourt, T. S. (2015). The youth readiness intervention for war-affected youth. *Journal of Adolescent Health, 56*, 606–611.

O'Callaghan, P., Branham, L., Shannon, C., Betancourt, T. S., Dempster, M., & Mcen, J. (2014). A pilot study of a family focused, psychosocial intervention with war-exposed youth at risk of attack and abduction in northeastern Democratic Republic of Congo. *Child Abuse and Neglect, 38*(7), 1197–1207. doi:10.1016/j.chiabu.2014.02.004.

O'Callaghan, P., McMullen, J., Shannon, C., Rafferty, H., & Black, A. (2013). A randomized controlled trial of trauma-focused cognitive behavioral therapy for sexually exploited, war-affected Congolese girls. *Journal of the American Academy of Child and Adolescent Psychiatry, 52*(4), 359–369. doi:10.1016/j.jaac.2013.01.013.

O'Callaghan, P., McMullen, J., Shannon, C., & Rafferty, H. (2015). Comparing a trauma focused and non trauma focused intervention with war affected Congolese youth: A preliminary randomised trial. *Intervention, 13*(1), 28–44. doi:10.1097/WTF.0000000000000054.

Peltonen, K., & Punamäki, R.-L. (2010). Preventive interventions among children exposed to trauma of armed conflict: A literature review. *Aggressive Behavior, 36*(2), 95–116. doi:10.1002/ab.20334.

Peltonen, K., Quota, S., El-Sarraj, E., & Punamäki, R.-L. (2010). Military trauma and social development: The moderating and mediating roles of peer and sibling relations in mental health. *International Journal of Behavioral Development, 34*(6), 554–563. doi:10.1177/0165025410368943.

Persson, T. J., & Rousseau, C. (2009). School-based interventions for minors in war-exposed countries: A review of targeted and general programmes. *Torture, 19*(2), 88–101.

Qouta, S. R., Palosaari, E., Diab, M., & Punamäki, R.-L. (2012). Intervention effectiveness among war-affected children: A cluster randomized controlled trial on improving mental health. *Journal of Trauma Stress, 25*(3), 288–298. doi:10.1002/jts.21707.

Rubio, D. M., Schoenbaum, E. E., Lee, L. S., Schteingart, D. E., Marantz, P. R., Anderson, K. E., … Esposito, K. (2010). Defining translational research: Implications for training. *Academic Medicine, 85*(3), 470–475. doi:10.1097/ACM.0b013e3181ccd618.

Slone, M., Shosani, A., & Lobel, T. (2013). Helping youth immediately after war exposure: A quasi-randomized controlled trial of a school-based intervention program. *Journal of Primary Prevention, 34*(5), 293–307. doi:10.1007/s10935-0013-0314-3.

Staples, J. K., Atti, J. A. A., & Gordon, J. S. (2011). Mind-body skills groups for posttraumatic stress disorder and depression symptoms in Palestinian children and adolescents in Gaza. *International Journal of Stress Management, 18*(3), 246–262. doi:10.1037/a0024015.

Tol, W. A., Komproe, I. H., Jordans, M. J., Gross, A. L., Susanty, D., Macy, R. D., & de Jong, J. T. (2010). Mediators and moderators of a psychosocial intervention for children affected by political violence. *Journal of Consulting and Clinical Psychology, 78*(6), 818–828. doi:10.1037/a0021348.

Tol, W. A., Komproe, I. H., Jordans, M. J. D., Vallipuram, A., Sipsma, H., Sivayoka, S., … de Jong, J. T. (2012). Outcomes and moderators of a preventive school-based mental health intervention for children affected by war in Sri Lanka: A cluster randomized trial. *World Psychiatry, 11*(2), 114–122. doi:10.1016/j.wpsyc.2012.05.008.

Tol, W. A., Komproe, I. H., Jordans, M. J. D., Ntamutmba, P., Sipsma, H., Smallegange, E. S., … de Jong, J. T. V. M. (2014). School-based mental health intervention for children in war-affected Burundi: A cluster randomized trial. *BMC Medicine, 12*(56). doi:10.1186/1741-7015-12-56.

Tol, W. T., Komproe, I. H., Susanty, D., Jordans, M. J., Macy, R. D., & DeJong, J. T. V. M. (2008). School-based mental health intervention for children affected by political violence in Indonesia: A cluster randomized trial. *JAMA, 300*(6), 655–662. doi:10.1001/jama.300.6.655.

Tol, W. A., Song, S. Z., & Jordans, J. D. (2013). Annual research review: Resilience and mental health in children and adolescents living in areas of armed conflict—A systematic review of findings in low- and middle-income countries. *Journal of Child Psychology and Psychiatry, 54* (4), 445–460. doi:10.1111/jcpp.12053.

Wolmer, L., Hamiel, D., Barchas, J. D., Slone, M., & Laor, N. (2011). Teacher-delivered resilience-focused intervention in schools with traumatized children following the second Lebanon War. *Journal of Traumatic Stress, 24*(3), 309–316. doi:10.1002/jts.20638.

Woodside, D., Barbara, J. S., & Bernier, D. G. (1999). Psychological trauma and social healing in Croatia. *Medicine, Conflict, and Survival, 15*(4), 355–367. doi:10.1080/13623699908409477.

Zerhouni, E. (2003). The NIH roadmap. *Science, 302*(5642), 63–72. doi:10.1126/science.1091867.

Chapter 8
A Vision for Future Research from a Developmental Psychopathology Perspective

Keywords Positive outcomes · Resilience processes · Planned missing designs · Measurement timing · Multilevel structural equation modeling · Parallel process models · Latent change score modeling · Ecological resilience · Multilevel interventions

Returning to Fig. 3.1, despite the considerable activity in the area of program development for children exposed to political violence and armed conflict, the goal of conducting Tier 4 translational research has only just begun to be addressed. Therefore, we outline a road map for accomplishing this goal—one that reflects a developmental psychopathology perspective of youth developing in contexts of political violence.

Following a developmental psychopathology perspective, recommendations are organized by the tiers of the pyramid and aim to guide researchers at each tier to produce more information to be used by the subsequent tier. Although many of these recommendations can be applied across tiers of the pyramid, we will organize this discussion around how each tier of research can be improved to efficiently inform translational intervention and prevention efforts. These recommendations, described in greater detail below, suggest that at Tier 1 researchers should expand measurement to include outcomes beyond psychopathology—including positive outcomes, possible mediating variables, and risk and protective factors, while also including measures at multiple levels of the social ecology. Studies should be conceptualized to advance understanding of protective factors and resilience, as well as risk factors and psychopathology, and including assessments of multiple levels of the social ecology (Cummings & Valentino, 2015). At Tier 2, which aims to provide basic information about process-level mediators, we suggest at least two waves of data collection, including research designs that can allow for explicit tests of hypotheses about mediators and moderators. Moreover, a valuable direction would be to conduct such studies to follow up on hypotheses about mediators and/or moderators generated based on cross-sectional research (see Table 5.1). For longitudinal studies at Tier 3, we suggest a broadening of interests beyond between-subjects tests of mediators and recommend the use of multilevel structural equation modeling (MSEM) to test both within- and between-person processes. The use of MSEM also allows for modeling effects of the outer levels of the social ecology on youth development. Moreover, there is an urgent need to conduct this research in multiple new contexts worldwide, and to test a richer array of hypotheses about mediators and moderators, and a wider range of theoretical models. Finally, at Tier 4, we suggest utilizing intensive longitudinal designs to measure program processes as they are unfolding and including multiple levels of the social ecology in intervention efforts. In addition, there is an urgent test to accomplish and test prevention and intervention programs that are truly translational, based on program materials with a solid foundation in basic research, with rigorous tests of theoretical models for positive treatment outcomes, specifically, tests of mediators and moderators that provide bases for accounting for processes accounting for positive treatment outcomes.

At Tier 1, a first recommendation echoes recommendations of other prominent scholars in the field who have suggested measuring outcomes beyond psychopathology (e.g., Barber, 2009; Cairns & Dawes, 1996). From a developmental psychopathology perspective with the goal of informing translational programs (Cicchetti & Toth, 2006), we suggest researchers include both culturally relevant psychopathology constructs and positive outcomes. Factors that may shed light on resilience processes should also be assessed. The above review highlights significant variability across studies in youths' responses to political violence. This variability suggests the identification of relevant moderators will better inform for whom and under what conditions intervention and prevention programs should be targeted. In each context, identifying ways to strengthen individual-, family-, and community-level processes that set youth on a course of positive development will also be key to intervention and prevention efforts. Complementing the goal of reducing levels of psychopathology, this review also highlights the equally important goal of identifying constructs that promote positive youth development that could be targets for intervention.

Also at Tier 1, our second recommendation is to identify key mediating and moderating processes at multiple levels of the social ecology. Focusing too narrowly on individual processes or outcomes even in the initial research in a given area or conflict neglects the nature of how armed conflict impacts youth and the multiple environments in which they develop. Entire social ecologies are threatened in contexts of political violence. Governments falling cause dramatic shifts in the macrosystem; scarce resources strain relations across the exosystem; family separation and school disruption may tear at the sense of security provided by the microsystem. Given that development does not occur in a vacuum, even in basic cross-sectional studies, researchers should aim to assess factors outside of the youths' direct experience. This broader understanding of risk and protective factors may better inform future research and those intervening in emergency situations.

Despite calls for inclusion of multiple levels of the social ecology (e.g., home, school, and broader cultural influences), few studies actually measure variables at these levels much less account for them appropriately in their statistical models. One noted exception is a study by Cummings and colleagues (2013a) that used neighborhood-level crime data in a three-level model to understand child adjustment in Belfast. The results showed that individual-level exposure to political conflict was related to higher adjustment problems; moreover, neighborhood-level crime strengthened this relation. This finding suggests that the broader context in which youth exposure is occurring has important implications for individual-level processes. However, we recognize that data at this level may not be readily available in all contexts, especially in those communities where infrastructures have been destroyed or impaired. In these cases, researchers can use alternative methods of using individual-level data to capture these broader effects. For example, Christ and colleagues (2014) aggregated individual-level data regarding norms of inter-group contact at the neighborhood, region, and district levels to represent the contextual effect of contact on prejudice. Using seven different surveys across multiple countries, they showed that contact measured at the broader levels of the social ecology was related to less prejudiced attitudes. Therefore, modeling the influence of social-ecological effects on youth attitudes and developmental outcomes may be possible even in cross-sectional designs.

To balance our recommendations of including positive outcomes and other levels of the social ecology, we present a methodological strategy that may help given the time and participant burden limitations we all face. Planned missing designs allow researchers to assess more constructs with fewer items by randomly assigning participants to complete a subset of items on a given test or measure (Enders, 2010; Graham, Hofer, & MacKinnon, 1996). With the use of missing data designs, such as the multiple form design, researchers can measure more constructs from all of their participants by reducing the number of items of each construct completed by each person. Thus, planned missing designs reduce cost and burden on participants while measuring multiple constructs.

The ability to utilize planned missing designs grew out of widely available statistical packages that utilize full information maximum likelihood estimation and multiple imputation (Graham, Taylor, Olchowski, & Cumsille, 2006). The basic idea behind planned missing designs is that researchers can *plan* random missingness into their measurement procedure. For example, if researchers want to measure four constructs, each with 20 items, each participant would answer a total of 80 items. However, with planned missing designs, researchers can create multiple forms of their questionnaires such that each participant is only answering 60 questions, for example. Each form of the questionnaire would have some items from each of the four constructs, but not all. The different forms are then randomly assigned to participants. Because the data on each form is missing completely at random, maximum likelihood estimation and multiple imputation can be used to recover unbiased estimates of parameters of interest. There are several approaches to planned missing designs for missingness across items or across waves for longitudinal researchers. Readers are encouraged to read Enders (2010) and Graham et al. (2006) for full treatments of missing data approaches.

Planned missing designs may also enable researchers to balance cultural sensitivity with generalization across contexts. For example, in settings of political violence, researchers could use both locally derived measures and established measures of psychopathology and other outcomes. Assessing constructs in both ways would allow researchers to assess potential overlap in relevant constructs across contexts while also identifying differences. This more precise and inclusive data could help to potentially adapt existing interventions developed in Western culture (such as cognitive behavioral therapy) in culturally relevant ways. Thus, use of both sets of measures would allow for culturally sensitive assessment along with the ability to compare across contexts of conflict, with implications for intervention programs.

Although these recommendations apply across tiers of our pyramid, at Tier 2, the distinctive focus is on identifying mediating processes. To do so, we recommend researchers utilize at least two time-points of data collection to address research questions relating to between-person differences. An extensive body of work by Cole and Maxwell (Maxwell & Cole, 2007) suggests that assessing mediational processes with cross-sectional data can lead to biased findings. In particular, they found that, even in the case of complete mediation, the estimates of the direct effect and the indirect effect are biased in cross-sectional designs. As a follow-up to this work, Maxwell, Cole, and Mitchell (2011) showed that cross-sectional models are also biased in capturing indirect effects in the case of partial mediation. Even with large sample sizes, their work shows that the bias in cross-sectional models can either underestimate or overestimate the longitudinal indirect effects and total effects. Thus, the general recommendation when testing mediational models is to utilize longitudinal data.

At Tier 2, to assess mediation, researchers must also be aware of the timing of their measurements and how this timing corresponds with the pace of the unfolding processes of interest. Researchers should be aware of the assumptions of change they are making when choosing a particular analysis (Cole & Maxwell, 2009). For example, it is common for researchers to collect data in annual waves; however, the change pattern seen in the variable of interest may occur more quickly or more slowly. That is, if researchers measure violence exposure at time 1 and the mediator at time 2, the assumption is that the impact of that exposure is still lasting a year later, if measured annually. It may be the case that the relevant effect developed and returned to normal, or that it has yet to develop. The match between timing of exposure and measurement of outcomes could be related to the differences in prevalence rates of certain disorders seen across studies and contexts. Based on review of the available literature, researchers should be more precise about the patterns of change they expect and how these patterns inform the timing of assessments and analyses they choose to conduct. Thus, we recommend that researchers use modeling techniques to assess relations between variables that are sensitive to the time frame under which change is occurring for youth in settings of armed conflict.

We also derive recommendations for Tier 3 longitudinal studies of our road map from Cole and Maxwell's (2009) work related to risk research. To capture the true relation between the risk factor and developmental outcome, they point out researchers must be aware of the variability in onset of a given disorder, unknown time lag between the risk factor and the developmental issue, confounding of state and trait disorders, and changing nature of the developmental disorder (Cole &

Maxwell, 2009). Considering just the case in which all members of the population may have been exposed to the same war-related event at a given time, the onset of possible psychopathology or maladaptation may not occur at the same time for each person in the sample. Moreover, the duration of the given outcome or episode of disorder (e.g., major depressive episode) may vary between persons. These individual differences in relations between exposure and timing of onset and duration of developmental problems related to the stressor are not easily handled with commonly used longitudinal models such as multilevel modeling and latent growth curve modeling. Cole and Maxwell reference several other approaches including summary measures, such as using the area under the curve, which is a type of weighted average that includes both the maximum score for a given individual as well as the duration of the outcome. They also provide suggestions for additional analytical strategies to address the above mentioned issues with time-related characteristics of longitudinal studies. Thus, we recommend that researchers explicitly explore timing of assessment that accurately reflects their theoretical models and consider more appropriate statistical methods to understand the link between risk and youth development in settings of armed conflict.

Tier 3 studies are uniquely designed to be able to address person-oriented research (Bergman, von Eye, & Magnusson, 2006; Nesselroade & Molenaar, 2010). Using longitudinal research, we recommend researchers articulate questions that use appropriate statistical methods to examine *both* between- and within-person change processes. These directions are especially interesting for understanding developmental processes contributing to youth risk and resilience over time in contexts of political violence. Thus, Tier 3 longitudinal studies have the potential to go beyond between-person questions that dominate the literature on youth and armed conflict.

Research in this area to date, either explicitly or by default, tests mediation that occurs between people. These tests of between-person mediation have been utilized in Tier 3 across multiple contexts and assessing multiple mediator variables. For example, in Northern Ireland, Cummings and colleagues showed emotional insecurity mediates the relationship between exposure to violence and internalizing and externalizing symptoms (2013). In Sierra Leone, Betancourt, Agnew-Blais, Gilman, Williams, and Ellis (2010)'s stigma mediated the relationship between rape survival and depression. Typically tested with panel models or structural equation models, these analyses assess the effect of a given predictor variable X on outcome Y through mediator M. In the between-subjects design, these effects of X on M and M on Y are interpreted as relative to other people in the sample. Data is aggregated across multiple participants in the sample and assumes that the mediational process is the same for the whole population. However, in a within-subjects design, which requires multiple assessments of X, M, and Y, the indirect effect of interest is occurring within a person and individual differences in these effects can be predicted if significant variance in the effects is found. Although within-person models are emerging in the political violence and youth literature (e.g., Betancourt, McBain, Newnham, & Brennan, 2015; Cummings et al. 2013a, b, 2016; Merrilees et al., 2014a, b; Taylor, Merrilees, Goeke-Morey, Shirlow, & Cummings, 2014), tests of mediation with longitudinal data are still limited to between-person tests. For an example of tests of within-person models, see Cummings, Merrilees, Taylor, Goeke-Morey, & Shirlow, 2016).

Researchers studying youth exposed to political violence and armed conflict are likely interested in the assessment of multiple within-person changing processes. Two more commonly used approaches to assess these questions include latent growth curve modeling (Bollen & Curran, 2006) and multilevel models (Bryk & Raudenbush, 1992) which allow for the assessment of within-person changes in a single variable of interest. However, advanced modeling techniques, such as parallel process models and latent change score analysis, allow for the modeling of *multiple* changing variables of interest. Within structural equation modeling, parallel process models allow for the modeling of two or more variables with varying trajectories of change. Given the focus in the current review on the multiple variables within the social-ecological model that may affect youth development in contexts of political violence, researchers might be interested in within-person processes for both youth and their family members. For example, depending on review of the available literature and the investigators' conceptual model, one might be interested in whether within-person increases in youth depression following a war-related event are associated with within-person increases in depression for mothers. Although an extension of more commonly used within-person analyses, the parallel process model does have limitations that are addressed with other advanced approaches.

Latent change score modeling (McArdle & Hamagami, 2001) allows for the estimation of both the autoregressive component typically assessed in a cross-lagged panel models *and* within-person change assessed within latent growth curve modeling. First, cross-lagged panel models do not account for growth or decline in variables over time. Moreover, latent change score models also allow for the estimation of coupling parameters to assess links between the two (or more) changing variables. An advance over the correlations between latent changes in the parallel process model, these coupling parameters can estimate the time-dependent relations between the variables. For example, using bivariate latent change score modeling, Kouros, Quasem, and Garber (2013) found that adolescent anxiety symptoms predicted changes in depression symptoms *and* depression symptoms also predicted changes in anxiety symptoms. The benefit of using the latent change analysis is that the sequences of changes can be detected. In this case, the authors were able to determine that the sequence of changes truly does occur in both directions.

Given the strengths of other advanced approaches, however, we recommend researchers in the field of political violence and youth follow recent work by Preacher and colleagues (2010, 2011, 2015) that suggests disaggregating the between- and within-person effects using multilevel structural equation modeling (MSEM). This suggestion stems in part from the nested nature of the data collected from studies measuring multiple levels of the social ecology. Moreover, the intergroup nature of political violence and armed conflict naturally leads one to believe that observations within a study are not independent, but rather clustered by political, ethnic, or other relevant social categories. Experiences of and responses to political violence might also differ significantly from neighborhood to neighborhood of community to community. When we ignore this dependence in the data, we are violating assumptions of our tests leading to biased results. The second reason pertinent to our translational research goal is that failing to disaggregate the within- and between-level processes may give us incorrect information about at what level we should be intervening. The third reason is that MSEM allows for upper-level variables (e.g., levels representing outer levels of the social ecology) to be outcome variables.

MSEM is different from traditional approaches to multilevel modeling in that measurement error can be removed with the use of latent variables (instead of composite manifest scores) and it models the between- and within-person effects in the model as latent. Traditional multilevel modeling approaches to disaggregation of these effects rely on including grand-centered means of level 1 variables entered at level 2 and person-centered variables at level 1. This approach has been shown to be biased in overestimating the within-person effects. MSEM reduces this bias by providing more accurate estimates for different levels of effects (Preacher et al., 2010). Moreover, MSEM outperforms multilevel modeling approaches to multi-level mediation (Preacher et al., 2011). As Tier 3 research is crucial to identifying process-level mediators, it is of great importance that these effects be estimated without bias and with adequate estimation of the value of the indirect effect.

Across the studies in Tier 4, approaches typically targeted only one level of the social ecology (e.g., individual, family, and school). Yet the Tier 3 research pointed to the importance of "ecological resilience," that is, the notion that programs may be more effective if they address multiple levels of the social ecology (e.g., individual, family, and school) and should also be evaluated across levels (Tol, Song, & Jordans, 2013). More generally, the above review suggests intervention and pre-vention researchers should target more than one level of the social ecology (e.g., individual, family, and school) given the noted importance of "ecological resi-lience," or the idea that programs may be more effective if they address multiple levels of the social ecology. Effects of these interventions on multiple levels of the social ecology should also be evaluated. For example, to complement the valuable directions for school-based interventions, more emphasis needs to be placed on community interventions (Betancourt et al., 2013). The costs/benefits must be weighed when designing interventions at different levels of the social ecology that affect child adjustment; programs addressing only one level may limit the magni-tude, generalizability, or lasting nature of any effects. Although rarely attempted or accomplished, an ecological framework based on *multilevel* approaches to inter-vention appears to hold the most promise of substantial and long-term improve-ments in children's psychological well-being and adjustment (Betancourt et al., 2013).

Future translational research programs would be strengthened by greater engagement with basic research on the impact of armed conflict on children (see Tiers 1–3) and should consider targeting multiple levels of the social ecology. Moreover, consistent with the National Institute of Mental Health advice, prevention and intervention research holds particular (and largely untapped) promise for informing conceptual models and future basic research. That is, truly robust translational research will also include "bedside to bench" program evaluations that feedback to evaluate theoretically based explanatory processes (Cicchetti & Toth, 2006).

Researchers evaluating interventions should also be cognizant of measuring during the intervention. Exactly when interventions will have an effect on processes and outcomes is often unknown. Therefore, we recommend that researchers assess participants at multiple time-points during an intervention. For example, Hammack, Pilecki, and Merrilees (2014) examined daily assessments of variables such as feelings of empowerment, identity salience, and positive mood for Israeli, Palestinian, and American youth participating in an intergroup contact program. In addition to showing average-level differences in the groups over the two-week intervention, the results also indicated that Palestinian youth in a mutual differentiation condition of the contact program increased in empowerment through the program. In addition to questions about change in outcomes, multiple time-points during an intervention may also shed light on mediating processes. Utilizing multiple assessments during the intervention allows researchers to assess change (or lack thereof) in mediating processes targeted by the program. In the example above, assessment of the daily experience of the intervention program could also be used to examine day-to-day spillover processes. For example, if different topics are covered over multiple days during the program, researchers could examine changes in attitudes or emotions in days following those specific elements of the program.

Considering intervention and prevention approaches, latent change score modeling can also be beneficial in modeling dynamic processes in response to treatment (Ferrer & McArdle, 2010). Coupled with random assignment and the use of multiple assessments following the onset of intervention, latent change score modeling can be used to examine how change in one targeted process (e.g., intergroup contact) affects change in another process (e.g., out-group aggression) and how the strength of coupling between processes differs between treatments and control groups or among multiple different treatment approaches.

Although this road map outlines key recommendations for researchers working at each tier of the pyramid, with many advanced methodological points, we emphasize the importance of clear, accurate, underlying theory. That is, robust theoretical models that articulate specific predictions relating to timing and developmental change should guide study design, development, implementation, and evaluation. Without this theoretical foundation, statistical bases for adequately determining mediating and moderating processes may be inadequately articulated and/or justified. With these methodological advances, researchers may also be better positioned to test theoretical models against alternatives for greater conceptual clarity. Thus, rooted in theory, this road map outlines a number of possible ways to advance the study of youth and political violence and improve intervention efforts in settings of armed conflict.

References

Barber, B. K. (2009). *Adolescents and war*. Oxford: Oxford University Press.

Bergman, L. R., von Eye, A., & Magnusson, D. (2006). Person-oriented research strategies in developmental psychopathology. In D. Cicchetti & D. J. Cohen (Eds.), *Developmental psychopathology* (2nd ed., pp. 850–888). Hoboken, NJ: Wiley.

Betancourt, T. S., Agnew-Blais, J., Gilman, S. E., Williams, D. R., & Ellis, B. H. (2010). Past horrors, present struggles: The role of stigma in the association between war experiences and psychosocial adjustment among former child soldiers in Sierra Leone. *Social Science and Medicine, 70*(1), 17–26. doi:10.1016/j.socscimed.2009.09.038.

Betancourt, T. S., Borisova, I., Williams, T. P., Meyers-Ohki, S. E., Rubin-Smith, J. E., Annan, J., & Kohrt, B. A. (2013). Research review: Psychosocial adjustment and mental health in former child soldiers—A systematic review of the literature and recommendations for future research. *Journal of Child Psychology and Psychiatry, 54*(1), 17–36. doi:10.1111/j.1469-7610.2012.02620.x.

Betancourt, T. E., McBain, R. K., Newnham, E. A., & Brennan, R. T. (2015). The intergenerational impact of war: Longitudinal relationships between caregiver and child mental health in postconflict Sierra Leone. *Journal of Child Psychology and Psychiatry*. Advance online publication. doi:10.1111/jcpp.12389.

Bollen, K. A., & Curran, P. J. (2006). *Latent curve models: A structural equation perspective* (Vol. 467). Hoboken, NJ: John Wiley & Sons.

Bryk, A. S., & Raudenbush, S. W. (1992). *Hierarchical linear models in social and behavioral research: Applications and data analysis methods (1st ed.)*. Newbury Park, CA: Sage Publications.

Cairns, E., & Dawes, A. (1996). Ethnic and political violence—A commentary. *Child Development, 67*(1), 129–139. doi:10.1111/j.1467-8624.1996.tb01724.x.

Christ, O., Schmid, K., Lolliot, S., Swart, H., Stolle, D., Tausch, N., ... & Hewstone, M. (2014). Contextual effect of positive intergroup contact on outgroup prejudice. *Proceedings of the National Academy of Sciences, 111*(11), 3996–4000. doi:10.1073/pnas.1320901111.

Cicchetti, D., & Toth, S. L. (2006). Building bridges and crossing them: Translational research in developmental psychopathology. *Development and Psychopathology, 18*(3), 619–622. doi:10.1017/S0954579406060317.

Cole, D. A., & Maxwell, S. E. (2009). Statistical methods for risk-outcome research: Being sensitive to longitudinal structure. *Annual Review of Clinical Psychology, 5*, 71–96. doi:10.1146/annurev-clinpsy-060508-130357.

Cummings, E. M., Merrilees, C., Taylor, L. K., Goeke-Morey, M., & Shirlow, P. (2016). Emotional insecurity about the community: A dynamic, within-person mediator of child adjustment in contexts of political violence. *Development and Psychopathology,* doi:http://proxy.geneseo.edu:2108/10.1017/S0954579416001097.

Cummings, E. M., Merrilees, C. E., Taylor, L. K., Shirlow, P., Goeke-Morey, M. C., & Cairns, E. (2013a). Longitudinal relations between sectarian and nonsectarian community violence and child adjustment in Northern Ireland. *Development and Psychopathology, 25*(3), 615–627. doi:10.1017/S0954579413000059.

Cummings, E. M., Taylor, L. K., Merrilees, C. E., Goeke-Morey, M. C., & Shirlow, P. (2016). Emotional insecurity in the family and community and youth delinquency in Northern Ireland: A person-oriented analysis across five waves. *Journal of Child Psychology and Psychiatry, 57*(1), 47–54.

Cummings, E. M., Taylor, L. K., Merrilees, C. E., Goeke-Morey, M. C., Shirlow, P., & Cairns, E. (2013b). Relations between political violence and child adjustment: A four-wave test of the role of emotional insecurity about community. *Developmental Psychology, 49*(12), 2212–2224. doi:10.1037/a0032309.

Cummings, E. M., & Valentino, K. V. (2015). Development Psychopathology. In W. F. Overton & P. C. M. Molenaar (Eds.), *Theory and Method*. Volume 1 of the *Book of child psychology and developmental science*. (7th ed.), Editor-in-Chief: Richard M. Lerner. Hoboken, NJ: Wiley.

Enders, C. K. (2010). *Applied missing data analysis*. New York, NY: Guilford Press.

Ferrer, E., & McArdle, J. J. (2010). Longitudinal modeling of developmental changes in psychological research. *Current Directions in Psychological Science, 19*, 149–154. doi:10.1177/0963721410370300.

Graham, J. W., Hofer, S. M., & MacKinnon, D. P. (1996). Maximizing the usefulness of data obtained with planned missing value patterns: An application of maximum likelihood procedures. *Multivariate Behavioral Research, 31*(2), 197–218. Retrieved from http://search.proquest.com/docview/618808782?accountid=11072.

Graham, J. W., Taylor, B. J., Olchowski, A. E., & Cumsille, P. E. (2006). Planned missing data designs in psychological research. *Psychological Methods, 11*(4), 323–343. doi:10.1037/1082-989X.11.4.323.

Hammack, P. L., Pilecki, A., & Merrilees, C. (2014). Interrogating the process and meaning of intergroup contact: Contrasting theoretical approaches. *Journal of Community & Applied Social Psychology, 24*(4), 296–324.

Kouros, C. D., Quasem, S., & Garber, J. (2013). Dynamic temporal relations between anxious and depressive symptoms across adolescence. *Development and Psychopathology, 25*(03), 683–697.

Maxwell, S. E., & Cole, D. A. (2007). Bias in cross-sectional analyses of longitudinal mediation. *Psychological Methods, 12*(1), 23.

Maxwell, S. E., Cole, D. A., & Mitchell, M. A. (2011). Bias in cross-sectional analyses of longitudinal mediation: Partial and complete mediation under an autoregressive model. *Multivariate Behavioral Research, 46*(5), 816–841.

McArdle, J. J., & Hamagami, F. (2001). Latent difference score structural models for linear dynamic analyses with incomplete longitudinal data. *New methods for the analysis of change* (pp. 139–175). Washington, DC: American Psychological Association. doi:http://dx.doi.org/10.1037/10409-005.

Merrilees, C. E., Taylor, L. K., Goeke-Morey, M. C., Shirlow, P., & Cummings, E. M. (2014a). Youth in contexts of political violence: A developmental approach to the study of youth identity and emotional security in their communities. *Peace and Conflict: Journal of Peace Psychology, 20*(1), 26–39. doi:10.1080/10781910903088932.

Merrilees, C. E., Taylor, L. K., Goeke-Morey, M. C., Shirlow, P., Cummings, E. M., & Cairns, E. (2014b). The protective role of group identity: Sectarian antisocial behavior and adolescent emotion problems. *Child Development, 85*(1), 412–420. doi:10.1111/cdev.12125.

Nesselroade, J. R., & Molenaar, P. C. M. (2010). Analyzing intra-person variation: Hybridizing the ACE Model with P-technique factor analysis and the idiographic filter. *Behavior Genetics, 40*(6), 776–783. doi:10.1007/s10519-010-9373-x.

Preacher, K. J. (2015). Advances in mediation analysis: A survey and synthesis of new developments. *Annual Review of Psychology, 66*, 825–852. doi:10.1146/annurev-psych-010814-015258.

Preacher, K. J., Zhang, Z., & Zyphur, M. J. (2011). Alternative methods for assessing mediation in multilevel data: The advantages of multilevel SEM. *Structural Equation Modeling, 18*(2), 161–182. doi:10.1080/10705511.2011.557329.

Preacher, K. J., Zyphur, M. J., & Zhang, Z. (2010). A general multilevel SEM framework for assessing multilevel mediation. *Psychological Methods, 15*(3), 209–233. doi:10.1037/a0020141.

Taylor, L. K., Merrilees, C. E., Goeke-Morey, M. C., Shirlow, P., & Cummings, E. M. (2014). Trajectories of adolescent aggression and family cohesion: The potential to perpetuate or ameliorate political conflict. *Journal of Clinical Child and Adolescent Psychology, 13*(1), 1–15. doi:10.1080/15374416.2014.945213.

Tol, W. A., Song, S. Z., & Jordans, J. D. (2013). Annual research review: Resilience and mental health in children and adolescents living in areas of armed conflict—A systematic review of findings in low- and middle-income countries. *Journal of Child Psychology and Psychiatry, 54*(4), 445–460. doi:10.1111/jcpp.12053.

Chapter 9
Conclusion

Keywords Robust basic research · Iterative translational research · Developmental psychopathology · Limitations

There is an evident disconnect between basic research and applied efforts to promote the well-being of the one billion youth who are growing up in contexts of political violence and armed conflict worldwide. To this end, a major goal of this book was to argue for more robust basic research on developmental processes in these contexts. A second major goal was to argue for the bidirectional translation of research and applied practice in efforts to advance the well-being of affected youth. Informal and limited approaches to program development and evaluation leave many questions about how, why, and for whom particular prevention or intervention efforts may work, and, even more fundamentally, whether particular programs work at all.

In the absence of systematic efforts to construct a basic research foundation for translational work, it is unlikely cost-effective, efficacious, and scalable programs can be developed, or that generalizable principles for applying findings other contexts of armed conflict will be generated. Recent major reviews have primarily focused on the intervention literature, leaving out both systematic review of basic research (e.g., research described in terms of Tiers 1–3 in this review) and integration of basic and intervention research.

This book systematically brought together the multiple and valuable directions of previous studies on political violence and youth adjustment in a conceptual pyramid informed by the tenets of developmental psychopathology (Fig. 3.1). Thus, the value-added of this review is to bring together the multiple directions in research on political violence, armed conflict, and youth adjustment with clear recommendations for future research and practice.

Although the tiers closest to the pinnacle of our model (e.g., Tier 3) are potentially most pertinent to process-oriented program development and evaluation (e.g., Tier 4), elements reflected in each tier merit consideration in future prevention and intervention programs. That is, consistent with a developmental psychopathology

E.M. Cummings et al., *Political Violence, Armed Conflict, and Youth Adjustment*, DOI 10.1007/978-3-319-51583-0_9 perspective, work in each tier is mutually informative and synergistic with work in other tiers; the findings across the tiers should be systematically integrated to improve this field. More generally, the principles of a developmental psychopathology perspective (Cummings & Valentino, 2015) offer well-developed future directions for advances in the study of youth and armed conflict. For example, from this perspective, it would be advantageous to expand the range of outcomes and processes— including resilience and protective factors and processes—to further understand how youth respond to the unique challenges of political violence. Moreover, except to document that exposure to armed conflict poses risk for multiple forms of adjustment problems in children in selected contexts (e.g., Tier 1 research), there is limited evidence that the findings of basic research (e.g., Tiers 2 and 3) are considered in the development of intervention approaches. Thus, our pyramid model concretely depicts and encourages inclusive consideration of the contributions of research across all tiers with the aim of effective translation research.

Moreover, this book specifically highlights the importance of process-oriented, longitudinal research from a social-ecological perspective (e.g., Tier 3 research), and encourages interrelations between Tier 3 basic and Tier 4 process-oriented translational research. Following, a developmental psychopathology perspective, this review calls for translational research that is theory—and empirically guided and designed to test explanatory processes such as meditators and moderators. Beyond providing support for the efficacy of programs in changing outcomes, it is important for investigators to know how and why, and for whom and when, programs work, which provides firm bases for cumulatively building more beneficial, cost-effective, and generalizable intervention programs. Our roadmap for the future demonstrates the value and key recommendations within each tier of the pyramid, with concrete suggestions about how to move research forward. Ultimately, these recommendations aim to develop increasingly efficacious and effective intervention approaches.

This review also advocates for moving back and forth between basic and translational studies (e.g., bench to bedside, bedside to bench); this exchange may be iterative, with multiple strategies underway at the same time or progress though spirals rather than building blocks. We also recognize that given the urgency of this problem and the widespread nature of armed conflict, it may be necessary to move forward and test plausible theories of change through intervention with children affected by political violence, rather than waiting until the whole pyramid foundation is completed. However, it remains that all elements of the pyramid of evidence merit consideration in the development of intervention research and that the most definitive research, that is, Tier 3 longitudinal process-oriented research from a social-ecological perspective provides especially strong bases for theories of change or protection to be used in these cases.

Despite the many contributions of this book, several limitations merit consideration. Given the extensiveness of this literature, it was not possible to include all possible studies in the tables. Instead, we endeavored to sample among the strongest exemplars of each level of research, with the intention of reflecting the best of the current worldwide literature. Aiming for global diversity, the tables are rich and highly informative summaries of research design characteristics and main findings of cutting-edge studies representing the "state of the art" in how this research is conducted. While possibly some very good studies were excluded (e.g., non-English language, file drawer effect), the intent of our selection criteria was to ensure the tables included the most highly meritorious. In excluding non-English studies, we could have neglected to incorporate studies from certain conflicts and regions of the world. Thus, the tables provide an archival record of a significant body of the outstanding research on child development being done in many parts of the world affected by political violence and armed conflict at each tier of the pyramid.

Another limitation reflects the wide-ranging and complex literature on this issue. Few meta-analyses exist in this domain of inquiry, primarily because the literature is inconsistent, spotty, and somewhat disparate. Shortcomings are undoubtedly related to the extraordinary challenges of conducting high-quality research in current or former conflict zones, the difficulties of assessment comparing findings across diverse cultures. There are also substantive reasons for limited meta-analysis in this area. The reality is that contexts of political violence vary widely at all social-ecological levels, including the many possible theoretically driven mediators, moderators, and other explanatory variables. Thus, in addition to the fact that meta-analyses may not be feasible for many key questions, meta-analyses may inadvertently ignore many important elements of the context, or oversimplify tests of explanatory models.

In conclusion, this book presented a unique conceptual framework, grounded in the tenets of developmental psychopathology, to analyze the existing literature on youth adjustment in contexts of political violence and armed conflict. This analysis leads to a road map that suggests how to expand the range of analyzed outcomes and levels of the social ecology, as well as greater precision to estimating explanatory processes underling developmental outcomes. These recommendations for research design and statistical analysis may be applied across tiers of the pyramid. Without such advances and integrations of knowledge, findings from a process-oriented basic research approach and/or program evaluations of applied research are likely to remain qualified and potentially inconclusive. To increase the impact of our work, researchers should develop programs of investigation that are informed by developmental theory, basic and applied research, and should employ correspondingly complex designs and statistical methods. With the approach outlined by this review, it may be possible to truly advance understanding of the effects of political violence and armed conflict, and to develop strong practices for making positive and lasting differences in the lives of affected youth.

Reference

Cummings, E. M., & Valentino, K. V. (2015). Development psychopathology. In W. F. Overton &
P. C. M. Molenaar (Eds.), *Theory and method*. Volume 1 of the *handbook of child psychology
and developmental science* (7th ed.) (pp. 566–606). Editor-in-Chief: Richard M. Lerner.
Hoboken, NJ: Wiley.

Index

Note: Page numbers followed by f and t indicate figures an tables respectively

A
Adaptive behaviors, 59–60*t*, 61*t*, 84*t*
Adaptive processes, 76
Adaptive systems, 35
Afghanistan
    follow-up study of youth mental health, 73
    Tier 2 studies, 36*t*
    Tier 3 studies, 65–66*t*
Africa, 1, 14, 19
    Tier 1 studies, 22–23*t*
    Tier 2 studies, 36*t*
    Tier 3 studies, 59–65*t*
    Tier 4 studies, 83–84*t*
Armed conflict, 7, 15, 17, 18, 19, 29, 30, 98.
    See also Political violence
    American youth, 89
    defining, 2
    developmental processes, 52, 100, 101,
        108, 109
    risk and protective processes, 49
    social ecology, 82
    on youth adjustment, 21, 35, 57, 58, 76, 81,
        93
Asia, 14, 19
    Tier 1 studies, 23–26*t*
    Tier 2 studies, 36–46*t*
    Tier 3 studies, 65–68*t*
    Tier 4 studies, 84–88*t*

B
"Bedside to bench" program, 104, 108
Bosnia, 49
    Tier 1 studies, 26–27*t*
    Tier 2 studies, 46–47*t*

Bosnia and Herzegovina, 19, 20, 90, 91
    Tier 1 studies, 27*t*
    Tier 4 studies, 88*t*
Burundi, 74, 92
    Tier 3 studies, 59*t*
    Tier 4 studies, 83*t*

C
Cambodia, 19
    Tier 1 studies, 23*t*
Chechnya
    emergency education, 93
    Tier 2 studies, 47–48*t*
Chronosystem, 49
Cognitive appraisal, 46*t*, 49, 50, 51
Cognitive behavioral therapy, 83*t*, 84*t*, 86*t*, 87*t*,
    89, 91, 100
Cold War, 18, 19
Community acceptance, 59*t*, 60*t*, 61*t*, 62*t*, 74
Community-level factors, 73–74
Community violence, 69*t*, 70*t*, 71*t*, 72*t*, 75, 76,
    92
    nonsectarian, 69*t*, 70*t*, 71*t*, 74
    sectarian, 69*t*, 70*t*, 71*t*, 72*t*, 73, 74, 75
Competent functioning, 35
Consensus-based guidelines, 93–94
Coping strategies, 23*t*, 24*t*, 26*t*, 35, 50, 68*t*,
    69*t*, 86*t*
Coping style, 49, 50, 51
Croatia, 19, 58
    Tier 1 studies, 27–28*t*
    Tier 2 studies, 48*t*
    Tier 3 studies, 68–69*t*
    Tier 4 studies, 88*t*

© Springer International Publishing AG 2017
E.M. Cummings et al., *Political Violence, Armed Conflict, and Youth Adjustment*,
DOI 10.1007/978-3-319-51583-0

Cross-lagged panel models, 102
Cross-lagged path analyses, 74
Cross-sectional mediation and moderators
　　individual characteristics, 49–51
　　microsystem factors, 51–52
Cross-sectional research, 11, 15, 97
Cross-sectional studies, 49, 50, 98
Cultural differences, 21

D
Democratic Republic of the Congo, 89
　　Tier 4 studies, 83–84*t*
Demographic moderators, 19
Developmental contexts
　　need for understanding, 1
　　potential for resilience, 4
　　urgency of the study of, 3–4
Developmental psychopathology, 2, 19, 107,
　　109
　　assumptions, 2
　　framework for research on children, 12, 12*f*
　　as guiding model, 7–9
　　translational research, 7, 81
　　vision for future research, 97–104
Developmental theory, 8, 109
Dynamic developmental processes, central
　　concern, 7
Dynamic mediators, 19
Dynamic processes, 19, 57, 104

E
Ecological resilience, 103
Ecological systems theory, 49
Emotional security theory, 58, 75, 76–77
ERASE-Stress, 85*t*, 91
Ethnic-political violence, 2
Europe, 14, 19
　　Tier 1 studies, 26–28*t*
　　Tier 2 studies, 46–48*t*
　　Tier 3 studies, 68–72*t*
　　Tier 4 studies, 88*t*
Exosystem, 49, 88
Externalizing problems, 21, 29, 60*t*, 62*t*, 63*t*,
　　69*t*, 70*t*, 73, 74, 84*t*, 101

F
Family acceptance, 60*t*, 61*t*, 63*t*, 64*t*, 73, 76
Family support, 51
Family violence, 65*t*, 73
Four-tier "pyramid" model, 2, 11, 12*f*

Framework for research on children, 12, 12*f*

G
Guidelines. *See* Consensus-based guidelines

H
Herzegovina. *See* Bosnia and Herzegovina

I
Ideological commitments, 50
Individual characteristics, 93
　　in Tier 2 systems, 49–51
　　in Tier 3 systems, 58, 73
　　in Tier 4 systems, 89
Individuals' probabilities, 20–21
Indonesia, 90, 92
　　Tier 4 studies, 84–85*t*
Intergroup contact, 104
Internalizing problems, 20, 29, 47*t*, 48*t*, 60*t*,
　　61*t*, 62*t*, 63*t*, 69*t*, 70*t*, 73, 74, 81, 84*t*, 101
International Child Development Program, 90
Intervention-oriented search terms, 82
Ireland, Northern, 19, 73, 74, 75, 77, 101
　　Tier 1 studies, 28*t*
　　Tier 3 studies, 69–72*t*
Israel, 18, 19, 21, 49, 50, 91
　　Tier 1 studies, 24–25*t*
　　Tier 2 studies, 37–39*t*, 40–41*t*
　　Tier 4 studies, 85–86*t*
Israel and Palestine
　　Tier 2 studies, 39–40*t*, 41–42*t*
　　Tier 3 studies, 67–68*t*
Iterative translational research, 107

J
Jewish youth, 24*t*, 38*t*, 75
　　religious and non-religious, 50, 51

K
Kuwait, Tier 2 studies, 42*t*

L
Latent change score modeling, 102, 104
Latent growth curve modeling, 101, 102
Lebanon, 19, 43, 50
　　Tier 2 studies, 43*t*
　　Tier 4 studies, 86*t*
Limitations, 108
　　file drawer effect, 109
　　non-English language, 109

wide-ranging and complex literature, 109
Longitudinal designs, 11, 98
Longitudinal mediation, 57, 76, 82, 89, 97, 98, 100, 108. *See also* Tier 3 studies
Longitudinal research, 11, 51, 76, 101, 108
  developmental theory, 8
Longitudinal studies, 15, 97, 100, 101

M

Macrosystem, 49, 98
Major depressive episode, 101
Maladaptive processes, 7, 76
Maladjustment, 8, 9, 11, 13, 19, 20, 21, 29, 35, 51
Measurement error, 103
Measurement timing, 100
Mediation, 87*t*, 92, 100, 101, 102, 103
Mediators, 9, 11, 29, 94, 98, 100, 101, 108, 109
  dynamic mediators, 19
  in framework for research on children, 12, 12*f*
  individual characteristics, 49
  potential mediators, 52
  process-level mediators, 97, 103
  theoretically driven mediators, 109
  understanding, 15
  urgency of identifying, 94
Mesosystem, 49
Microsystem, 49
Moderators, 9, 11, 94, 97, 98, 108, 109
  demographic moderators, 19
  in framework for research on children, 12, 12*f*
  individual characteristics, 49
  modifiable moderators, 19
  post hoc moderators, 93
  process-oriented moderators, 11, 29
  psychological moderators, 52, 76
  social moderators, 52
  understanding, 15
  urgency of identifying, 94
Mother-child dyad, 37*t*, 38*t*
Multilevel interventions, 103
Multilevel modeling, 101
Multilevel structural equation modeling (MSEM), 97, 102, 103

N

National Institute of Mental Health, 103
Nepal, 19, 92, 93
  Tier 1 studies, 25*t*
  Tier 2 studies, 43–44*t*

Tier 4 studies, 86*t*

O

Out-group aggression, 104

P

Palestine, 19
  Tier 1 studies, 26*t*
  Tier 2 studies, 44–46*t*
  Tier 3 studies, 66–67*t*
  Tier 4 studies, 87*t*
  youths' activities, Intifada, 21
Parallel process models, 102
Parent-child relationship, 44*t*, 51
Person-oriented research, 58, 75, 101
Planned missing designs, 99
Political violence, 7, 8, 15, 17, 18, 19, 58, 101, 102, 108. *See also* Armed conflict
  defining, 2
  family intervention, 89
  maladjustment, 35
  in Northern Ireland, 74
  and psychological problems, 20, 21
  repercussions, 29
  school intervention, 90, 91
  social ecologies, 98
  translational research, 81
  and youth adjustments, 29, 50, 51, 52, 57, 73, 76
  and youth development, 49, 50, 77, 93, 101
Positive outcomes, 57, 97, 98, 99
Posttraumatic stress disorder (PTSD), 14, 18, 19, 20, 92
Posttraumatic stress symptoms (PTSS), 91, 92
Prevention and intervention studies, 81–82, 89
  individual characteristics, 89
  microsystem factors (*see* Tier 4 microsystem factors)
Primarily cross-sectional designs, 11
Primarily longitudinal designs, 11
Process-level mediators, 97
Process-oriented program, 107, 108, 109
  social-ecological perspective, 108
Process-oriented research
  developmental psychopathology, 7
  Tier 3 research (*see also* Tier 3 studies), 57
Process-oriented tests, 2
Protective processes, 35
  and risks, 8, 49, 52, 77
Psychological constructs, 98
Psychosocial interventions, 83*t*, 90, 91, 92
PsycINFO, 13, 82

R

Randomized clinical trials (RCTs), 81–82
Regulatory processes, 58
Resilience, 19, 20, 29, 76, 97, 98, 101, 108
    ecological resilience, 103
    processes, 4, 103
Risks, 20, 29, 30
    and protective processes, 8, 49, 52, 77
Robust basic research, 107, 109
Rwanda, Tier 1 studies, 22*t*

S

School-based intervention approach,
    advantages, 93
Sierra Leone, 58, 73, 74, 89, 101
    Tier 2 studies, 36*t*
    Tier 3 studies, 59–64*t*
    Tier 4 studies, 84*t*
Social ecology, 58, 98, 99
    multiple levels of, 35
Social identity theory, 75
Social support, 23*t*, 42*t*, 46*t*, 59*t*, 62*t*, 64*t*, 65*t*,
    69*t*, 76, 83*t*, 85*t*, 90
    acceptance and, 52
Social-ecological contexts
    individual characteristics, 49–51
    microsystem factors, 51–52
Social-ecological model, 8
    four-tier "pyramid" model, 2
South Africa, 19
    Tier 1 studies, 22*t*
Sri Lanka, Tier 4 studies, 87–88*t*
Structural equation modeling (SEM), 58

T

Teacher-delivered programs, 90
Three-level model, 98–99
Tier 1 studies, 17, 22–28*t*
    in Africa, 22–23*t*
    in Asia, 23–26*t*
    in Europe, 26–28*t*
    historic research, 17–18
    limitations, 29
    methodological strategy, 99
    planned missing designs, 99
    recent studies, 19
    search strategy for identifying, 13–15
    three-level model, 98–99
    translational programs, 98
    youth outcomes, 19
Tier 2 studies
    in Africa, 36*t*
    in Asia, 36–46*t*
    in Europe, 46–48*t*

identifying mediating processes, 100
individual characteristics, 49–51
microsystem factors, 51–52
Tier 3 studies
    in Africa, 59–65*t*
    in Asia, 65–68*t*
    between-subjects design, 101
    beyond the microsystem, 74
    in Europe, 68–72*t*
    individual characteristics, 58, 73
    longitudinal models, 101
    microsystem factors, 73–74
    multiple levels of social ecology, 75
    person-oriented analyses, 75–76
    person-oriented research, 101
    risk factor and developmental issue,
        100–101
    social-ecological perspective, 57
    within-person change, 75–76, 102
Tier 4 microsystem factors
    family, 89–90
    school, 90–93
Tier 4 studies
    in Africa, 83–84*t*
    in Asia, 84–88*t*
    in Europe, 88*t*
Translational research, 1, 2, 81
    developmental psychopathology, 7
    fostering cogent scientific bases for
        prevention and intervention, 8–9
    goal of, 12
Trauma-focused cognitive-behavioral therapy,
    83*t*, 84*t*, 89
Traumatized youth, 4

U

Uganda, 19, 20, 93
    Tier 1 studies, 22–23*t*
    Tier 3 studies, 64–65*t*

V

Violence exposure, 21, 22*t*, 100
    community, 28*t*

W

War-affected youth, 50
Web of Science, 13, 82
Within-person change, 75–76
World War II, 17

Y

Young evacuees, strain, 18
Youth adjustment, 13, 18, 19, 20, 29, 35, 76,
    89, 107, 109

antisocial behavior, 74
emotional insecurity, 73
political violence on, 49, 50, 51, 57
regulators of, 51
role of community and family factors, 76, 77

social-ecological effects, 99
Youth living, attention, 1
  need for understanding, 1
  potential for resilience, 4
  urgency of the study of, 3–4

CPSIA information can be obtained
at www.ICGtesting.com
Printed in the USA
LVHW082044140219
607571LV00012B/251/P